DICTIONARY OF PUBLIC HEALTH PROMOTION AND EDUCATION

Terms and Concepts

Second Edition

NAOMI N. MODESTE
TERI S. TAMAYOSE
Foreword by Helen Hopp Marshak

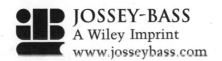

JOSSEY-BASS
A Wiley Imprint
www.josseybass.com

Published by Jossey-Bass
A Wiley Imprint
989 Market Street, San Francisco, CA 94103-1741   www.josseybass.com

Jossey-Bass books and products are available through most bookstores. To contact Jossey-Bass directly call our Customer Care Department within the U.S. at 800-956-7739, outside the U.S. at 317-572-3986 or fax 317-572-4002.

Jossey-Bass also publishes its books in a variety of electronic formats. Some content that appears in print may not be available in electronic books.

Library of Congress Cataloging-in-Publication Data

Dictionary of public health promotion and education : terms and concepts / Naomi N. Modeste, Teri S. Tamayose, editors.— 2nd ed.
    p. ; cm.
    Rev. ed. of: Dictionary of public health promotion and education / Naomi N. Modeste. c1996.
    Includes bibliographical references and index.
    ISBN 0-7879-6919-2 (alk. paper)
    1. Health education—Dictionaries. 2. Health promotion—Dictionaries. 3. Health education—Societies, etc.—Directories. 4. Health promotion—Societies, etc.—Directories.
    [DNLM: 1. Health Education—Dictionary—English. 2. Health Education—Directory. 3. Health Promotion—Dictionary—English. 4. Health Promotion—Directory. 5. Public Health Practice—Dictionary—English. 6. Public Health Practice—Directory. WA 13 D5535 2004]   I. Modeste, Naomi N. II. Tamayose, Teri S., 1960- III. Modeste, Naomi N. Dictionary of public health promotion and education.
    RA440.5.M634 2004
    613'.03—dc22   2004013525

Printed in the United States of America

PB Printing   10 9 8 7 6 5 4 3 2 1   SECOND EDITION

CONTENTS

FOREWORD

Helen Hopp Marshak

This dictionary was developed for professionals in the field of health promotion and health education and in related professions. It identifies a wide range of terms and health and professional organizations commonly used by health educators and public health professionals, although it is not meant to be exhaustive. The contents reflect the *process* of health promotion and education rather than disease-specific terminology. Key terms used in related public health disciplines, such as epidemiology, health administration, biostatistics, environmental health, and behavioral sciences, were included because health educators are ordinarily expected to be familiar with these areas in their practice. Terms relevant to the four settings of health promotion and education—community, workplace, primary care, and school—are emphasized.

This dictionary was originally prompted by our graduate students' request for a reference list of terms that they could understand and employ consistently in their professional reading and writing. Conversations with other health educators confirmed the need for such a guide. The first edition has been used by public health professionals in both academic and practice settings and has proved to be a valuable resource for arriving at a common understanding of terms frequently encountered by health educators.

This second edition expands on the core health education terminology presented in the first edition. Emphasis was placed on delineating terms related to theories and models commonly used by health educators, including planning and evaluation models, as well as key methods and strategies used by health educators that define the scope and nature of the profession. Newly emerging areas, such as health informatics and computer-assisted instruction, are also included.

Although it is impossible to present definitions that everyone will agree with, every attempt was made to cross-reference terms with a wide variety of key sources in health education. The references cited in the text and listed at the end of this guide were used as resource materials for deciding on definitions. Suggestions for further reading follow the References.

It is hoped that this expanded guide will be useful to professionals in health promotion and education and their colleagues.

ACKNOWLEDGMENTS

This book grew out of concerns shared by a number of our graduate students for a list of terms that can be used as a quick reference guide. The reports of the 1990 and 2000 Joint Committee on Health Education Terminology provided additional motivation for this work.

We wish to thank Helen Hopp Marshak, a colleague in the Department of Health Promotion and Education, Loma Linda University, School of Public Health, for writing the Foreword, sharing resources, and giving valuable suggestions for several entries.

We also acknowledge the help of the individuals who reviewed the manuscript and made suggestions and corrections, particularly Joyce W. Hopp, Tom Schiff, Larry Olsen, and Brick Lancaster. Finally, recognition goes to editor Andy Pasternack and his associates at Jossey-Bass for their valuable suggestions, encouragement, and support throughout this project. We take responsibility for any weaknesses or omissions.

INTRODUCTION

This dictionary provides definitions of terms and concepts frequently used in public health promotion and health education, written in a manner that can be easily comprehended. Many of us in the field of health education have learned a great deal about significant health-related concepts but use terminology that is not necessarily found in any one text. This work is an attempt to bring together a number of these terms under one cover for easy access.

Our intent was to include the terms most widely used by a large number of people in the various disciplines of public health, particularly health education and promotion, and also to include terms from related disciplines with which health educators need to be familiar.

Many books and journal articles, especially more recent articles, have been searched for new terms that appeared since the first edition of this book. These terms, along with most of those featured in the first edition, have been brought together, defined, and arranged in a dictionary format. Our objective is that anyone who uses this resource, whether student or health professional, will be able to look up a definition without wading through scores of pages of books and journal articles. No attempt, however, was made to include all of the terms ordinarily used, and we made a particular effort to exclude disease-specific terms; so this work is by no means exhaustive. It was not an easy task to select which resources to include as references and which to omit, as the same terms were referenced by multiple authors. Some important references may have been unintentionally omitted.

The definitions vary in length, as is to be expected given that some terms are simpler and more easily defined while others call for more detail and perhaps even examples. Many entries have been cross-referenced to show how they relate to one another.

Some terms might not meet strict health education and health promotion definitions, but keep in mind that health education relies on many other disciplines, including epidemiology, environmental health, behavioral sciences, and theories of learning.

This dictionary can be used as a companion to health education texts and courses of study by both undergraduate and graduate students, as well as in their preparation for the CHES examination. It can also serve as a source of reference for practicing health educators, faculty, and other health professionals involved in health education and promotion.

The dictionary is divided into two parts. Part One lists the selected terms alphabetically. This style was chosen because it provides a simple method of finding the entries and reflects the style of most dictionaries. If you wish to look up *bioterrorism,* for example, you'll find it under *B.* If you want to find a definition for *comprehensive health education* or *community health,* turn to *C* and look for them alphabetically. Do not become frustrated if a term you are searching for is not included; although many new terms have been included, as stated previously, it is not the purpose of this dictionary to include all the terms that you might find appropriate to health education and promotion.

Part Two lists, in alphabetical order, several professional and voluntary health organizations and agencies of which students and practicing health educators need to be aware. Like the list of terms in Part One, this section is not exhaustive. Key organizations are listed, including mailing addresses and Web sites where information can be acquired.

A major objective in compiling this book was to keep it financially accessible to students while at the same time including sufficient terminology and associations for organizations to improve health education information and promote health literacy.

Dictionary of Public Health Promotion and Education

PART ONE

Terms

A

Abstinence

Refraining from the use of drugs, alcohol, tobacco, and other substances or habits that tend to harm the body. May also refer to refusing to engage in sex behaviors that may put individuals at risk for early pregnancy or diseases such as HIV/AIDS and other sexually transmitted infections (STIs).

Abstinence Violation Effect (AVE)

Part of Marlatt and Gordon's 1985 model of the relapse process involving a cognitive-emotional reaction that includes (a) guilt from relapsing and engaging in an undesired behavior (e.g., smoking) after quitting smoking or changing the behavior (e.g., smoking cessation), which is discrepant from the new self-image (e.g., a nonsmoker); and (b) an attribution that the relapse episode was due to personal weakness. This usually results in perceptions of decreased self-efficacy in considering readopting a desired health behavior (Cormier, 2002; Parks, Anderson, & Marlatt, 2001; Shiffman et al., 1996). In addition to smoking, AVE can be experienced among binge eaters (Grilo & Shiffman, 1994) and people with other addictive disorders. See *Relapse Prevention*.

Access to Health Care

The ease with which individuals or groups of people obtain health care or health services in a given community. Individuals with reliable health insurance, a regular provider for health care, and higher income may have easier access to quality health care, because of their ability to pay for service, while those with inadequate health insurance and low socioeconomic status may have limited access to health care (Bodenheimer, & Grumbach, 2002; McKenzie, Pinger, & Kotecki, 2002; U.S. Department of Health and Human Services, 2000). Health educators look at access to health care in terms of transportation, location of facility, hours of operation, cost and financing (including health insurance), and social, ethnic, language, and geographical concerns that may help or hinder individuals in obtaining health care.

Accreditation

A process carried out by educational and medical institutions and organizations for quality assurance. Accreditation attempts to ensure quality of care in medical facilities such as hospitals, and academic quality in educational institutions such as colleges and universities. The process is conducted by an external accrediting body and is based on predetermined standards to certify that the requirements for academic or health care excellence are met either permanently or for a period of time.

Acculturation

The process of making modifications in one's own culture to incorporate behavior patterns, traits, or new ideas from another culture. Acculturation takes place when a person moves to a new culture and is being socialized into that culture.

Action Plan

A list of detailed steps to be taken to accomplish a specific goal, followed by an outline or timetable designed to accomplish each step listed. See *Timeline*.

Administrative Assessment

A review of prevailing policies, resources, and circumstances in communities or organizations to determine which of them help or hinder the development of a health promotion and education program. The procedure includes resource assessment, setting a timetable for activities, and budgeting (Green & Kreuter, 1999). It focuses on the assignment of the resources and responsibilities for implementing and evaluating the proposed program or project.

Adverse Health Effect

Any change in body function resulting from unsafe levels of exposure to substances such as chemicals or pollutants in the environment that can be detrimental to human health or might lead to disease or some type of health problem.

Affective Domain

A category for classifying learning objectives that emphasize feeling and emotion, from the simplest outcomes to the most complex: personal interests, attitudes, values, appreciation, and methods of adjustment. Knowledge is more effective in shaping health-related behavior when combined with affective associations (Anderson & Krathwohl, 2001; Butler, 2000).

Example: (*learning objective stated in the affective domain*) "By the end of this session, the student will be able to verbalize personal feelings about taking medication for hypertension."

Affective Learning

Learning associated with beliefs, self-worth, appreciations, and values during which learners are emotionally and actively involved in the learning experience and in relating to others. It can be opposed to cognitive learning (Himsl & Lambert, 1993). See *Affective Domain* and *Cognitive Learning*.

Agent

An organism or object that transmits disease from the environment to the host or from one person to another. "The cause of the disease or health problem, the factor that must be present in order for the disease to occur" (McKenzie, Pinger, & Kotecki, 2002, p. 595). In health education and promotion, the term may also be applied to persons such as village and community health workers, community elders, teachers, and health educators who communicate health messages or act as channels through which ideas and innovations are transmitted to potential consumers. See *Host*.

Examples: The human immunodeficiency virus (HIV), which causes acquired immunodeficiency syndrome (AIDS); the tick that carries the virus for Colorado tick fever; and the mosquito that carries the infection for malaria are all etiological agents.

Air Pollution

The contamination of air by pollutants (smoke, ash, dust, pollen, acid condensates, etc.), including carcinogenic substances that cause discomfort to people and can be hazardous to health when breathed.

Alma Ata Declaration

A statement released by the World Health Assembly at the International Conference of Primary Health Care meeting in Alma Ata, Kazakh Soviet Socialist Republic (now Kazakhstan), on September 12, 1978. Its aim was to commit all member countries of the World Health Organization (WHO) to the incorporation of lifestyle and behavioral factors and improvement of the environment into the principles of health for all by the year 2000. Primary health care was the principal thrust of the declaration, but it also incorporated community participation in an effort to protect and promote the health of all the people of the world (Bunton & Macdonald, 1992). The declaration affirmed that health is a fundamental human right that should be made attainable for all people and that individuals have a right to participate in planning their health care.

At-Risk Groups

Groups or populations who, due to certain common existing economic, social, and environmental factors or behavioral characteristics, may be prone to a certain disease or condition.

Examples: Coal miners or coal workers; parenteral drug users; homosexuals and heterosexuals with multiple partners; employees in a clinical laboratory; persons practicing anal intercourse

Attitudes

Favorable or unfavorable evaluative reactions or dispositions toward a situation, a person, or a group, as expressed in one's beliefs, feelings, or behavior (Rajecki, 1990). An attitude that a person holds toward hypertension, for example, will influence behavior intentions with respect to the problem.

Example: "I like high-fat foods."

Because attitudes may be either positive or negative, there are times when helping people change attitudes is as important as helping them change behavior.

B

Baseline Measures

Data collected prior to a program implementation and used for comparing measures before and after the program to determine the effectiveness of the program or new intervention.

Example: Blood pressure measurements may be taken at a specific time (baseline); then a program of exercise and nutrition is implemented, and blood pressure measurements are taken again about six weeks into the program and compared with the baseline measurements to determine if the intervention is effective.

Behavior

Any observable response to a stimulus or an action that has a "specific frequency, duration and purpose, whether conscious or unconscious" (Green & Kreuter, 1999, p. 503). Internal responses such as thinking or feeling may be inferred from observable behavior.

Behavior may also refer to how people react with one another as well as their environment and can be considered as a product of heredity, culture, and environment. Behavior can be both positive (beneficial) and negative (harmful). Health educators encourage positive behaviors (U.S. Department of Health and Human Services, 2000).

Examples: Mothers in a given community breast-feed their babies from birth through the first six months without introducing other foods and liquids, Carolyn exercises thirty minutes a day five times a week to maintain her weight.

Behavior Modification

One of the major approaches to learning and behavior change in health education, based on principles of respondent and operant learning, involving changing an individual's response by manipulating the environment—specifically, stimuli of a behavior or reinforcement of a behavior. Behavior modification may also be considered a coping strategy.

Behavior modification uses the following approach (Martin & Pear, 1992):

1. Identify the problem.
2. Describe the problem in behavioral terms.
3. Select target behaviors that are measurable.
4. Identify antecedents and consequences of the behavior.
5. Formulate behavioral objectives.
6. Devise and implement a behavioral change program.
7. Plan and execute an evaluation program.

Example: Using the behavior modification approach to reduce overeating would involve the following steps. First, specify the behavioral goal or goals: Reducing the number of snacks or amount of food eaten throughout the day. Second, observe and record the target behavior: Keep a count of the number of times food is eaten during a twenty-four-hour period or a food diary recording types and amount of food eaten at each meal. Third, identify what cues the problem behavior and attempt to alter these stimuli: If overeating while watching television, avoid eating while watching television. Fourth, identify and substitute new thoughts and behaviors for old, undesirable eating habits. Fifth, identify and alter reinforcers for overeating. Sixth, evaluate behavior modification strategies, reward yourself, and if necessary move on to another behavior problem. Recent applications of behavior modification have added the additional step of relapse prevention strategies for encouraging people to maintain their desirable behavior changes (Foreyt, Goodrick, Reeves, & Raynaud, 1993; Marcus et al., 2000; Shiffman et al., 1996).

Behavioral Diagnosis
Systematic analysis and delineation of specific health-related behavioral problems that can likely affect the outcome of a health program, based on the PRECEDE/PROCEED Model of health education program planning

(Chiang, Huang, & Lu, 2003; Green & Kreuter, 1999). See *PRECEDE/ PROCEED Model.*

Behavioral Epidemiology

The study of individual health-related behaviors and habits in relation to health outcomes, taking into account the role of individual behavior in causing and maintaining disease. Also includes health promotion and disease prevention research and evaluation focusing on health behaviors (Catania & Dolcini, 2002; Owen & Crawford, 2001; Sallis, Owen, & Fotheringham, 2000).

Example: An examination of smoking behavior and later health outcomes, such as the incidence of lung cancer

Behavioral Health

The promotion of health by emphasizing the role behavior plays in achieving or maintaining health. Also involves the application of behavioral and biomedical science knowledge and techniques through a variety of activities to maintain health and prevent disease (Kaplan, 1990). Behavioral health is relevant to health education and focuses on promoting health among people who are currently healthy.

Behavioral Health Care Services

Health services provided to people with mental health and substance abuse problems, emotional and behavioral health disorders, and addictions.

Behavioral Intention

The likelihood that a person will engage in a given behavior, based on the attitudes and subjective norms held by the person (Farley & Stasson, 2003; Masalu & Åstrøm, 2003; ÅRajecki, 1990; Schwarzer & Renner, 2000). Originally derived from the theory of reasoned action, which later became the theory of planned behavior (Ajzen, 1991).

To predict whether or not a person will perform a certain action, you can simply ask the person. A more precise measure of likelihood may be obtained by asking the person to indicate his or her probability of carrying out the action. See *Theory of Planned Behavior* and *Theory of Reasoned Action*.

Example: An individual may be asked to indicate the likelihood that he or she might abstain from sex within the next year, as follows:

I intend to abstain from sex within the next year.

Likely —|—|—|—|—|— Unlikely

Or the person may be asked to estimate the likelihood of his or her abstaining from sex within the next year in percentage points:

There is a ____ percent chance that I will not have sex within the next year.

Behavioral Medicine

Behavioral science knowledge and techniques that are relevant to the understanding of physical health and illness and the application of this knowledge and these techniques to prevention and treatment, as well as rehabilitation. Behavioral medicine is concerned with various issues that may influence health and illness, including the environment in which one lives, socioeconomic status, family dynamics, and other social factors (Gonder-Frederick, Cox, & Ritterband, 2002; Keefe, Buffington, Studts, & Rumble, 2002; Pruitt, Klapow, Epping-Jordon, & Dresselhaus, 1998; Whitfield, Weidner, Clark, & Anderson, 2002).

Behavioral Objective

A statement describing precisely what the learner will be doing as a result of a learning experience, expressed in measurable terms. Also called a performance, educational, or learner objective.

Example: "By the end of the program, 60 percent of seminar participants will commit themselves to establishing a smoke-free environment at their workplace within six months."

Belief

A proposition or statement emotionally or intellectually accepted as true by a person or group.

Benchmarking

Evaluating and measuring performance by comparing programs, organizations, or systems to similar programs, organizations, or systems as part of continuous quality improvement.

Biofeedback

A therapeutic method or technique used to increase awareness of a person's own physiology. On the basis of feedback from the body, one may be able to control physiological processes such as blood pressure or stress symptoms. Small changes in visual and auditory signals are used to make a person aware of bodily processes of which he or she was previously unaware, and the person eventually learns to control the biological system on the basis of this information (Hermann, Blanchard, & Flor, 1997).

Biofeedback focuses on the biological systems that are beyond conscious control but are acting in a way that impairs the individual's performance, thereby contributing to stress-related diseases. In the biofeedback process, the individual first becomes aware of any faulty response, then is guided by the feedback signal to control the response, and learns to transfer this control to everyday situations.

Biofeedback is used to teach people how to relax in stress management programs and for the control of hypertension, anxiety, insomnia, and other stress-related disorders (Kaplan, Sallis, & Patterson, 1993).

Bioinformatics

The application of statistical and computer technology to store, retrieve, and analyze biological and health data for research and the improvement of health and behavioral sciences (Hunter, 2004; Watanabe, 2004). The National Institutes of Health Bioinformatics Definition Committee (2000), chaired by Michael Huerta, released the following definition: "Research, development, or application of computational tools and approaches for expanding the use of biological, medical, behavioral, or health data, including those to acquire, store, organize, archive, analyze, or visualize such data" (p. 1).

Biological Monitoring

The constant surveillance or measuring of chemical or biological substances in water, air, and soil for quality and characteristics or agents that may cause serious injury or death within populations. Also, testing blood, hair, breath, or urine to determine if individuals were adversely exposed to substances such as lead.

Biomedical Science

Science concerned with human (or animal) biology and disease, along with prevention, diagnosis, and treatment of disease.

Bioterrorism

The unlawful release of toxic agents or biological agents such as bacteria or viruses into the environment (including food and water) that can adversely affect humans, animals, or plants, with the intent of harming people.

Block Grant

Financial aid received by state governments from the federal government to assist cities and counties in community development, social services, education, and health. An example is the Preventive Health and Health Services Block Grant administered by the Centers for Disease Control and Prevention (CDC), which provides federal funding to all fifty states and to U.S. territories for combating chronic diseases and for health education and prevention services.

    The federal government has used block grants as incentives to help the states and counties develop health services in a variety of programs, such as tuberculosis control, dental health, mental health, home health, maternal and child health, primary care, and alcohol and drug abuse prevention.

Features distinguishing block grants from other forms of federal assistance include authorizing of funds for a wide range of activities within broadly defined functional areas; giving recipient states discretion in identifying problems, designing programs, and allocating resources; and minimizing administration in financial reporting, planning, and other federal requirements. Block grants afford recipients a degree of financial security.

Brainstorming

A technique used in a group situation to generate as many ideas about a particular question, topic, or problem as possible in a given (usually brief) period of time. Group members are encouraged to express their thoughts spontaneously, postponing evaluation and criticism of ideas until after the brainstorming session is over.

C

Capacity Building

The building of an infrastructure for the delivery of health promotion programs. Includes the allocation of resources and the formation of partnerships to support and achieve change; the development of multiple stakeholders and information systems for sustaining initiatives and programs; and the coordination and management of community programs for change. Also refers to programs that are designed to build a healthier community and are either community-based or institutionally based.

Capitation

A plan of payment for health care providers whereby a fixed amount is paid by an insured individual to cover a set of services over a period of time, and institutional providers are also paid a fixed amount for persons served. This method is characteristic of certain health maintenance organizations.

Carrier

A person or animal that harbors a specific infectious agent but not the disease and serves as a source of infection (Benenson, 1990; Chin, 2002); also known as a *healthy carrier.*

Example: A person may carry the typhoid bacillus, the infectious agent for typhoid, and although showing no symptoms of the disease or of becoming sick with typhoid, pass it to others through direct (person-to-person) contact or indirect contact (in contaminated food or water or via the urine).

Case Control Study

A study comparing a group of people with a diagnosed or specified disease or problem with one or more groups who do not have the same diagnosis or specified disease. Typically, case control studies are carried out retrospectively, because they often assess past exposure among cases (individuals with the disease) and controls (those without the disease).

Case Study

An account of a problem situation that includes sufficient information to enable meaningful discussion of contributing factors, possible preventive measures, and alternative solutions.

A case study approach to health promotion and education provides documentation of experiences to help others in the profession, particularly new entrants to the profession. For examples of case studies, see McConnell (1998) and Breckon (1997).

Catchment Area

An area defined within a population that is served by a health program or a health agency or institution selected on the basis of factors including geographical boundaries, site accessibility, and population distribution. All individuals residing in a catchment area would be eligible for the services or programs offered by the institution or agency.

Certification

A process by which a quasi-governmental agency or association grants recognition or licensure to a person who has met certain qualifications specified by that agency. The National Commission for Health Education Credentialing (NCHEC) is the association responsible for granting certification to health educators. Health educators who receive certification become Certified Health Education Specialists (CHES). See *Certified Health Education Specialist (CHES);* see also *National Commission for Health Education Credentialing (NCHEC)* in Part Two.

Certified Health Education Specialist (CHES)

A person who has met all of the requirements established by the National Commission for Health Education Credentialing (NCHEC) and has received recognition (a certificate) as a health educator who has met the qualifications of training and experience to practice health education and has been successful in the examination or grandfathered in by the commission. The acronym CHES after a health educator's name indicates professional competency in the seven areas of responsibilities of a health educator. See *Certification* and *Credentialing;* see also *National Commission for Health Education Credentialing (NCHEC)* in Part Two.

Chain of Command

In management, a hierarchy in which supervisors have authority over the individuals they supervise and a clear determination is made as to who reports to whom.

Change Advocate

An individual, such as a health educator or leader, who strongly supports and encourages change within his or her organization, cause, or personal philosophy.

Change Agent

An individual or organization whose role is to assist other individuals or groups in identifying and dealing with issues and to guide others in a direction considered desirable. A change agent can also function in diagnosing or assessing health concerns as well as in planning and evaluation.

Health educators function as change agents when they work with people and encourage or influence them to make desirable changes, such as giving up smoking during pregnancy.

Chronic Disease

A condition or health problem affecting a person for a prolonged period of time that may result in permanent residual disability. A chronic illness may persist and become acute, ending in a crisis or death. Such a disease is marked by long duration or frequent recurrence and may require long periods of intervention or supervision.

Examples: Hypertension, diabetes mellitus, chronic respiratory problems, chronic pain, congenital heart disease

Coalition

A group of organizations in a community united to pursue common goals and specific problems. Organizations and groups join to address community issues, combining talents and resources to tackle new problems and accomplish broader goals than any one group or individual can manage (Rowitz, 2001). They remain free to enter and leave at will.

A coalition may include several health agencies working together for a common good. In health education and promotion, coalitions are usually formed to deal with specific health problems in defined communities. Coalition building is essential to community-based health intervention programs and leads to increased community awareness and commitment. In addition, coalitions help address political issues that may prevent well-planned programs from being implemented. In recent years, coalitions for smoke-free societies have been quite active, especially in California (Bracht, 1990). For additional reading on coalitions, see Green and Kreuter (1999).

Examples: The Community Antidrug Coalitions of America in Alexandria, Virginia, is a national coalition organization whose aim is to create safe, drug-free communities for kids. The Community Coalition for Substance Abuse Prevention and Treatment of Los Angeles was formed to improve the quality of life especially among low income families in South Central Los Angeles, to reduce the high concentration of liquor stores, and to empower youth to be advocates for a healthier drug-free community.

Codependency

The circumstance of individuals who are "dependent on making other people dependent on them as a means of self-validation" (Seaward, 1994, p. 97) and exhibit behaviors similar to addictive behaviors. A codependent person shows evidence of addiction to another person's addiction problems.

Usually, the relationship between the persons is close, such as parent-child or husband-wife.

Example: Children of alcoholic parents may become codependent on their parents' addiction and problems.

Cognitive-Behavioral Therapy

A treatment approach that combines cognitive and behavioral principles to change thoughts or behavior. Cognitive-behavioral therapy may be effective in interventions for abstinence from smoking (Hall, Munoz, & Reus, 1994), panic disorder (Laberge, Gauthier, Cote, Plamondon, & Cormier, 1993), and chronic headache (James, Thorn, & Williams, 1993).

Cognitive Dissonance

Conflict between a person's beliefs and the person's behavior, based on Festinger's theory of cognitive dissonance (Aronson, 1992; Carkenord & Bullington, 1993; Cooper, 1992; McMaster & Lee, 1991).

Example: A person may know and believe that chewing tobacco can cause mouth cancer but goes ahead and chews anyway. The person can try to dissolve the dissonance either by altering the perception of the risk or by giving up chewing.

Cognitive Field Theory

A theory used mainly to explain how human behavior is learned, according to which learning should not only be identified with cognition but should also be purposeful, explorative, and innovative.

Cognitive Learning

Learning associated with how individuals process information. The mental process or thought process of acquiring, perceiving, and organizing information. The ability to memorize, understand, and apply information or knowledge to life situations, intellectual performance, problem solving, and behavior change.

Cohort

A group of people identified by certain characteristics or statistical factors, such as age, and followed or observed at different points over a long period of time from exposure to a disease to the development or manifestation of the disease (Powers & Knapp, 1990; Vogt, 1993).

A cohort is a "component of the population born during a particular time period and identified by period of birth so that the characteristics of this group at different points in time can be identified." The term is also "more generally used to describe any group of people who are followed or traced over time" (Bunton & Macdonald, 1992, p. 226).

Examples: A group of coal miners aged twenty-five to thirty-five years being followed up for possible development of lung disease; children born after the Chernobyl accident followed up for twenty years to measure radioactive iodine in the thyroid or possible radiation-induced cancers; a group of teenagers who began smoking in 1990 followed up over a twenty-year period for possible development of lung cancer

Collaboration

Working together, teaming up, sharing responsibilities, or joining forces to create community intervention programs to promote health and effect behavior change or achieve goals. Several organizations may formally commit themselves to work together in developing a specific project or in accomplishing a mission. Collaboration involves shared decision making and allocation of resources (Austin, 2000). It promotes healthy working relationships and creative solutions to problems or needs, builds bridges in a community, and pools resources to effect change.

Examples: School nurses may collaborate with other community service providers in an effort to meet multiple health needs of students; one nation may join forces with another nation for medical and epidemiological

research (as in the case of AIDS, affecting countries worldwide); health educators may collaborate with communities for promoting primary health
care and health education needs (Cowley, 1994; Handler, Schieve, Ippoliti,
Gordon, & Turnock, 1994; Ritchie, 1994; Statham, 1994).

Collective Bargaining

"The formal process of negotiating and administering a written signed
agreement between labor and management. Collective bargaining usually
covers wages, working conditions, and fringe benefits, and the agreement,
once signed, has the force of law" (Breckon, 1997, p. 310).

Communication

The process by which messages are transferred through a channel to a
receiver and information is shared with other individuals. Communication
can be written, verbal, and nonverbal. See *Communication Channel*.

Communication Channel

The mechanism that carries information from its source to its destination.
Communication channels may include interpersonal (face-to-face) communication, broadcasting (radio or television), and print (newspapers, mag-
azines, posters, pamphlets, flyers). See *Communication*.

Community

A geographical area considered as a unit, a group of people held together
by common interests or goals and a "sense of identity," or a collection of
people characterized by membership (a sense of identity and belonging)
or common values, language, rituals, ceremonies, needs, or history
(Wurzbach, 2002).

A community may also be a group of people experiencing the same
need, regardless of geography. A community of migrant workers scattered
across the country might share the same identifiable needs.

Health educators recognize the concept of community as an integral
part of community health education and health promotion. In most

instances, the community can be defined as a geographical unit, such as a county, city, town, or neighborhood.

Community Assistance Panel

A panel consisting of members eighteen years of age and older from the community and health organizations to discuss and share health information and community concerns and issues about the exposure to hazardous substances and how they might have been exposed or could be exposed.

Community-Based Care

Health and social services including health promotion and education that are provided in communities or places of residence to ensure easy access to health care, the provision and maintenance of health, and the prevention of disease and disability.

Community-Based Participatory Research

Research based in a community and for the community that involves the community in its planning and implementation. The approach is one of equitable collaboration with community members in all the stages of planning, collecting and analyzing the data, and disseminating findings of the research endeavor. It's a cooperative approach that educates and empowers community members to have some control over the research process and overall, to improve health conditions within their specific communities (Levy, Baldyga, & Jurkowski, 2003; Minkler & Wallerstein, 2003).

Community Capacity

The ability of a community or group to identify, implement, strengthen, and sustain collective efforts to promote community interests. In health education, it is the ability to effect change or improve the public's health by collaborative efforts and partnerships of groups, communities, and ag·ncies (Goodman et al., 1998).

Community Development

The attempt to organize and stimulate local initiative and leadership in a community to encourage change. The emphasis in community development is on local, self-determined efforts. Community development is process-oriented and emphasizes the development of skills and abilities conducive to social and health improvement. Community development ideas have been used by health educators in many countries in the world to improve health, family planning, childhood nutrition, and agriculture. See *Community Organization.*

Example: A community development program intended to help mothers grow vegetables to supplement family nutrition was established by allotting garden plots to families in the village and teaching the people simple gardening techniques.

Community Empowerment

"A social action process in which individuals and groups act to gain mastery over their lives in the context of changing their social and political environment" (Wallerstein & Bernstein, 1994, p. 142). Conceived as a health-enhancing strategy, community empowerment focuses on both individual and community change, encouraging people to listen to each other and dialogue with each other to discover new ways of looking at health problems and solutions (Israel, Checkoway, Schulz, & Zimmerman, 1994).

Community empowerment includes the ability of people actively working together to gain understanding and control over personal, political, social, and economic forces in a community. Individuals and community organizations collectively use their skills and resources in a long-term commitment to assume more control over processes of defining problems and setting priorities in an effort to enhance health and quality of life (Fetterman, 2002).

Community Forum

A public meeting in which key community residents and representatives review various perspectives on a particular issue—for example, community health. Such forums are broad-based and encourage community involvement and participation.

Community Health

Health promotion and education directed at populations rather than individuals, involving the science and art of promoting health, preventing disease, and prolonging life through organized community effort (Lowis, 1992).

Community Health Education

Education focused on the improvement of health and prevention of diseases within a community. Intergroup relationships, value patterns, communication resources, community organizations, policymaking, strategic planning, and related methods, including theoretical frameworks, are used to educate and mobilize community members to take actions that will enhance health and prevent disease.

Community health education is the application of a variety of methods that result in the education and mobilization of community members in action for resolving health issues and problems that affect the community. These methods include group process, mass media, communication, community organization, organizational development, strategic planning, skills training, legislation, policymaking, and advocacy. It is also defined as "a theory-driven process that promotes health and prevents disease within populations" (2000 Joint Committee on Health Education Terminology, 2001, p. 5).

Example: The Pawtucket Health Heart Program in Rhode Island is a communitywide cardiovascular disease prevention program employing a variety of community-based interventions, targeting worksites, restaurants, schools, grocery stores, individuals, small groups, and the community at large in an effort to reduce the incidence of heart disease through screening, health education, and counseling programs directed toward risk factors such as high blood pressure, elevated cholesterol, cigarette smoking, obesity, and sedentary lifestyle (Hunt et al., 1990; Lasater et al., 1991).

Community Health Educator

A health professional trained in health education or public health who works in a community setting, applying a variety of methods that result in the education and mobilization of community members in actions for resolving health issues and problems that affect the community.

"A community health educator is a practitioner who is professionally prepared in the field of community/public health education who demonstrates competence in the planning, implementation, and evaluation of a broad range of health promoting or health enhancing programs for community groups" (1990 Joint Committee on Health Education Terminology, 1991, p. 105). See *Community Health Education.*

Community Norm

"Specific rules of behavior that are agreed upon and shared within a culture to prescribe limits of acceptable behavior" (Tischler, 1993, p. 51).

Community Organization

The process whereby community members join forces in working together to identify needs, set objectives, and take definitive action consistent with local values to develop plans for community improvement, be it in health or other matters. Health educators and health advocates may play a vital role in organizing community members and groups to join forces for child and family violence reduction or injury control.

Community Participation

Involvement of individuals and groups in the community in events, planning, advocacy, community development, health promotion, and decision making in a variety of prevention programs. Inviting and allowing the community to participate in learning and the provision of services related to health care and health outcomes, as well as in research development.

Competitive Learning

A form of learning, or learning process, in which learners compete with each other (or with themselves) to achieve certain standards of learning. It is the opposite of *cooperative learning.* See *Cooperative Learning.*

Complementary and Alternative Health Practices

Practices for health maintenance, health enhancement, and disease prevention that employ natural substances and certain self-care methods and therapeutic approaches that are not considered conventional. Therapies may include the use of certain herbs, massage therapy, acupuncture, and vitamins. In 1998, the National Center for Complementary and Alternative Medicine was established at the National Institutes of Health to support research in this area of practice.

Compliance

In public health and health promotion, the act of following the advice of a physician or other health care worker in a prescribed therapeutic or preventive regimen. Also referred to as *cooperation* or *adherence.*

Example: Joyce just learned that she is at high risk for coronary heart disease, and she has been given a weekly exercise regimen as a preventive measure. She complies by performing the exercises as prescribed.

Comprehensive Health Education

Multidimensional programs planned and carried out by local, county, state, or federal governmental agencies for the purpose of maintaining, reinforcing, or enhancing people's health, health-related skills, and health attitudes and practices, coordinating education, services, and environment.

Comprehensive health education is not limited to governmental agencies. Private organizations may provide comprehensive programs for a smaller community such as a workplace or school.

Examples: A comprehensive program at the local level is the Homeless Prenatal Program (HPP), established in a San Francisco family shelter in

1989. This program provides comprehensive prenatal services to homeless pregnant women, aimed at improving their pregnancy outcomes and transforming their lives. Included in the program are good mothering techniques, prenatal care, peer support, supportive work environment, and job skills training (Ovrebo, Ryan, Jackson, & Hutchinson, 1994). The Healthy Beginnings program focuses on the development among children up to five years old in the social, emotional, physical, and cognitive domains. This program is part of the Comprehensive Health Education for Life (CHEF) skill-building program.

Comprehensive School Health Education

The planned, coordinated provision of school health services, a healthful school environment, and health instruction (education) for all learners (and staff) in a school setting in which each component complements and is integrated with the others in the total scope of the body of knowledge unique to health education. Comprehensive school health education addresses all the dimensions of health and is aimed at improving student health and academic achievement (Brindis, 1993; Satcher & Bradford, 2003; Seffrin, 1990; Wilson & Schuler, 2002).

Comprehensive school health education covers a variety of learning experiences appropriate to schoolchildren. It involves health education carried out in a school setting to improve health attitudes and practices and to enhance and maintain health. Some programs also offer health education opportunities for family and community members (Cleary, 1993b; Waller & Goldman, 1993).

Comprehensive school health education aims at protecting and promoting the health and well-being of students before entering kindergarten through grade 12 (Butler, 2000; 2000 Joint Committee on Health Education Terminology, 2001). Although qualified teachers certified to teach in the state, together with licensed and registered nurses, provide much of the health education in schools, school health educators are also playing a vital role in the school system in many states. In some instances, health educators may serve as health consultants, especially for the health education curriculum.

Comprehensive School Health Instruction

"The development, delivery, and evaluation of a planned curriculum, preschool through 12, with goals, objectives, content sequence, and specific classroom lessons" (1990 Joint Committee on Health Education Terminology, 1991, p. 106). Content areas may include community health, consumer health, environmental health, family life and sexuality, mental and emotional health, injury prevention and safety, nutrition and weight problems, substance use and abuse, personal health, and the prevention and control of disease.

Comprehensive School Health Program

"An organized set of policies, procedures, and activities designed to protect and promote the health and well-being of students and staff, which has traditionally included health services, healthful school environment, and health education. It should also include . . . guidance and counseling, physical education, food service, social work, psychological services, and employee health promotion" (1990 Joint Committee on Health Education Terminology, 1991, p. 105).

Computer-Assisted Instruction

The use of computers to teach and furnish students with information. Aimed at providing students with opportunities for putting what they learn into practice, this type of instruction can also be employed in evaluating students' achievement.

Conflict Resolution

A process used to resolve disputes, requiring the ability to seek understanding and solutions despite differences in ideas, social background, culture, and points of view. Success in conflict resolution requires being able to control emotional responses, recognize personal biases, and consider other perspectives on an issue.

Construct Validity

"Conformity to theoretical expectations of relationships between a previously untested measure and other variables" (Powers & Knapp, 1990, p. 25). Also, the degree to which survey instruments measure what they are intended to measure and the variables being tested are correlated for the survey's purpose.

Consumer Health

Decisions that individuals make regarding the purchase and use of health products, information, and services that are available in the marketplace and can affect their health positively or negatively. The focus of consumer health is on the importance of consumers' health care and the impact of health information being communicated to them (Moorman, 2002).

Consumer health also includes individual actions that are self-motivated and self-initiated, such as the purchase of aspirin for headache or the selection of a physician.

Content Analysis

A technique for systematically and quantitatively analyzing the content of communication, whether verbal, written, or pictorial. The technique can be used to determine the prevailing social values of a group or society.

Content Outline

A written guide that indicates the detailed process to be used for each activity listed in a lesson plan. The outline relates to the listed objectives of the lesson plan and usually incorporates the entire lesson. Health educators often use a content outline when teaching specific health education topics to target groups at schools, colleges, universities, and community settings.

Content Validity

"The subjective determination of validity, usually by some sort of expert judgment" (Powers & Knapp, 1990, p. 164). It reflects the degree or extent to which items or questions on a test or questionnaire are representative of the subject (Vogt, 1993).

In determining content validity, items on an instrument (questionnaire or test) should come from each content area to be measured. A review of the literature helps establish content validity by providing comprehensive information about the topic. See *Validity*.

Example: A health educator is the principal investigator in AIDS-related research among teenagers, looking at their knowledge, attitudes, and beliefs. The questionnaire developed for this survey should include questions on each area of interest.

Contributing Factor

Any behavioral or environmental element that has a potential for affecting health behaviors. Contributing factors can be categorized as motivators, enablers, or reinforcers. See *Enabling Factor* and *Reinforcing Factor*.

Cooperative Learning

People teaching each other, sharing each other's knowledge, or working together to achieve specific learning goals. Cooperative learning is being used successfully by teachers and researchers in many levels of education. In public health, especially community health education, cooperative learning can be effective as peers teach peers about health. For example, teenagers can be taught the ill effects of and alternatives to tobacco smoking, and these same teens can then teach other teens by sharing what they have learned. Or if health information is passed to a group regarding environmental health concepts, group members may cooperatively share this information with their peers so that they can work cooperatively to improve their immediate environment. Cooperative learning is the opposite of competitive learning (Cartwright, 1993; Huber, 2003; Slavin, Hurley, & Chamberlain, 2003). Instead of competing, students share information they have learned in the classroom with other students; they work together on projects and make cooperative decisions on issues. See *Competitive Learning*.

Coordinated School Health Program

"An organized set of policies, procedures, and activities designed to protect, promote, and improve the health and well-being of students and staff, thus improving a student's ability to learn. It includes . . . comprehensive school health education; school health services; a healthy school environment; school counseling; psychological and social services; physical education; school nutrition services; family and community involvement in the school; and school-site health information for staff" (2000 Joint Committee on Health Education Terminology, 2001, p. 6).

Coping

The constantly changing cognitive and behavioral efforts that individuals make in attempts to manage specific external or internal demands that they have appraised as taxing or exceeding their resources.

Most authors in the field of stress and coping recognize two primary categories: problem-focused coping and emotion-focused coping. Problem-focused coping involves taking focused action to eliminate a problem or change a situation. Emotion-focused coping includes efforts to modify impaired emotional functioning in the face of threat without trying to change the problem or situation directly.

Example: A person diagnosed with cancer (the stressor or problem) may make attempts to deal with the problem using problem-focused coping to deal directly with the cancer (seeking treatment, changing diet) and emotion-focused coping to deal with distress (attending a support group).

Cost-Benefit Analysis

A measure or evaluation of the cost of an intervention relative to the benefits it yields, usually expressed as a ratio of dollars saved or gained for every dollar spent on a program. In cost-benefit analysis, program costs and benefits are stated in monetary terms to ascertain whether the benefits exceeded the cost, even though it is difficult to place a dollar value on all program outputs (Breckon, 1997; Siegel & Doner, 1998; Windsor, Baranowski, Clark, &

Cutter, 1994). The potential benefits in dollars saved are divided by the cost of the intervention to provide the cost-benefit ratio.

Example: A health educator carries out a cost-benefit analysis on the cost of starting and maintaining a smoking cessation program for pregnant smokers. The cost per person enrolled will be calculated. On the benefit side, costs associated with the risk factor (smoking) include a reduction in absenteeism from work due to illness and lower medical costs to employers.

Cost-Effectiveness Analysis

A measure or evaluation of the cost of an intervention relative to its impact, usually expressed in dollars per unit of effect. Cost-effectiveness analysis is aimed at determining the cost and effectiveness of an activity to ascertain the terms of the degree to which the objectives or outcomes are attained.

Cost-effectiveness analysis may also involve comparing programs to determine which one provides the greatest level of effectiveness at least cost; the service that provides the lowest cost-per-unit benefit is the most cost-effective.

Credentialing

A formal process applied to ensure that persons practicing in a profession meet minimum standards of professionalism and practice. Through credentialing, health education professionals identify and provide verification of special skills and competencies. Standards of credentialing in heath education are based on seven broad areas of responsibilities and competencies for entry-level health educators (Clark, Ogletree, McKenzie, Dennis, & Chamness, 2002; Cleary, 1993a; Girvan, Hamburg, & Miner, 1993; Livingood et al., 1993; Mail, 1993). See *Entry-Level Health Educator.*

The credentialing process carried out by the National Commission for Health Education Credentialing (NCHEC) includes an examination of persons who have obtained a bachelor's degree or master's degree in public health. If successful, the credentialed health educator becomes a Certified Health Education Specialist (CHES). Certification is renewed annually through continuing education credits, and recertification takes place every five years.

Credentialing encourages professional growth, development, and lifelong learning through professional development opportunities. See *Certification* and *Certified Health Education Specialist (CHES);* see also *National Commission for Health Education Credentialing (NCHEC)* in Part Two.

Criterion Validity

The accuracy of a test or measurement to predict a behavior or attribute of opposite dimension or another criterion in the future. For example, the Graduate Record Examination (GRE) has criterion validity if the scores predict a person's academic performance in graduate school.

Cross-Sectional Study

A study of the effects of a disease or condition and its outcome in individuals or groups at a specific point in time. Inferences about the differences between age groups, for example, are based on observations of people of different ages measured at the same moment. Cross-sectional designs help describe variables of interest and their distribution patterns in the population.

Example: In the Health and Nutrition Examination Survey (HANES), a sample of people was carefully selected to represent the U.S. population. The people were interviewed about their health and habits, such as the prevalence of hypertension and the average daily intake of dietary fat. Comparisons are then made between groups of persons of different age, gender, race, and so forth.

Cultural Competence

The capability to understand and respect cultural values, mores, attitudes, beliefs, ideas, behaviors, and customs that are different from one's own and the ability to respond effectively to those differences when planning, implementing, and evaluating health education programs across cultures. Health educators increasingly face situations that necessitate working in communities of diverse cultural backgrounds and need to be able to promote health in multicultural settings. They should make an effort to maintain an awareness of the cultural differences that exist and to work effectively in a culture with values and beliefs that may differ from their own (Huff & Kline, 1999; Luquis & Pérez, 2003).

Culture

The sum of values and traditional ideas transmitted to individuals in a community over a period of time, or patterns of behavior acquired or learned and transmitted by human groups. Culture includes how people behave, think, and communicate their values, ideas, customs, attitudes, beliefs, and mores (Huff & Kline, 1999; Tischler, 1993).

The concept of culture is important to public health and particularly health education because the cultural background, including mores, norms, and ideologies, of an individual or a community has a profound effect on the response to health education and health promotion. When designing health education programs, cultural understandings and values must be recognized in order to make the programs appropriate for the particular group.

Curriculum Guide

A written plan containing detailed information regarding health education programming. It describes the goals, philosophy, scope, and sequence of a health education program.

D

Database

A collection of information stored in a computer, where it can be retrieved for future use.

Deductive Learning

A methodology in which facts and premises are assumed to be accurate and a conclusion is drawn based on these known truths; the opposite of *inductive learning.* In the health education field, deductive learning is characterized chiefly by memorization of certain health facts presumed to lead to a change in health behavior.

Example: Adolescents taught that flossing their teeth will prevent decay and early loss of teeth acquire the facts and technique of flossing and carry out the behavior with the hope that the desired result will occur (Bedworth & Bedworth, 1992).

Delphi Technique

A sampling method used to obtain an expert opinion without a face-to-face meeting. A series of self-administered questionnaires are mailed to a number of experts, opinion leaders, or informants to establish, for example, which participants would be appropriate for a particular program or which health education program should be implemented in a community. After three or four rounds of questioning, the results are polled, tabulated, and shared. The Delphi technique or process, unlike the nominal group process, allows participants to present their views impersonally and confidentially without overtly influencing the opinions of others (Sarvela & McDermott, 1993). This technique should be used only by trained professionals because although it is very effective with community groups, it can be viewed by some as manipulative. See *Nominal Group Process.*

Demography

The study of a population that is based on specific variables such as age, ethnicity, education, family income, employment, living arrangements, marital status, and religion, that can influence change within that population.

Dependent Variable

The presumed effect or outcome being measured, so called because it may *depend* on changes in the independent variable. In public health, health educators may assess the degree to which a risk factor (say, obesity) affects a health outcome (heart disease). The dependent variable (heart disease) varies with the independent variable (obesity) but may or may not be caused by it. The dependent variable is the variable of greatest importance to an investigator in a given study. See *Independent Variable*.

Examples: A researcher looks at the effects of participation in a weight reduction education program (independent variable) to see if there was a change or lowering of weight (dependent variable) in participants (Sarvela & McDermott, 1993). If you are studying the prevalence of heart disease among women aged fifty years and older, the presence of the disease is the dependent variable and age and gender are independent variables.

Determinants of Health

"Factors that significantly influence or have an impact on the health of individuals and communities" (Wurzbach, 2002, p. 5). These include genetic factors, income, poverty, environmental factors, political situations, unemployment and homelessness, education, social and economic circumstances including social exclusion and deprivation, workplace stress, established customs, and activities that affect the health status of individuals and communities (Gibbie, Rosenstock, & Hernandez, 2003).

Diagnosis

Identification of causes, characteristics, signs, and symptoms of a disease or condition. When used as an evaluative technique to analyze health issues, it is called *diagnostic evaluation.*

Diffusion Theory

A theory explaining the diffusion of something new (an innovation) among populations, groups, individuals, or social systems. Diffusion theory explains the pattern or rate of adoption of innovations by individuals or groups in a community—some persons may adopt new ideas immediately, others lag behind but adopt at some time, and some may not adopt at all (Howze & Redman, 1992).

Diffusion theory is a marketing principle used to explain the pattern of adoption of something new. There are four components to diffusion: (a) the innovation (a program or idea that is new), (b) the channels of communication by which the program or idea is exchanged among adopters or members of the group, (c) time, and (d) the setting or social system in which the innovation takes place (Schiffman & Kanuk, 1991; Valente, 1993).

Many health promotion programs are thought of as innovations among specific populations, and diffusion theory helps describe a pattern the population may follow in adopting the program (McKenzie & Jurs, 1993).

Example: Some people may hear of a nutrition education program to be implemented in their community and sign up to become involved without asking any questions. Others, more suspicious or less venturesome, wait until the program is under way to make sure it is useful; they probably wait to receive an invitation from someone who attended the first class before signing up and attending. Still others never become involved at all.

Disease

The failure of an organism to adequately or appropriately counteract stresses or stimuli, which can be biological, behavioral, or environmental, resulting in sickness or disability.

Disease Prevention

A process of reducing risk factors that lead to disease and disability, involving the promotion, preservation, and restoration of health as well as strategies to reduce suffering and early death in individuals or groups.

Dose-Response Relationship

The increase in an outcome measure associated with a proportionate increase of resources expended; a concept originating in the clinical trials of drugs but applicable to health promotion and education. In simple terms, the more material, money, human resource initiatives, and time put into a health promotion program, the greater the response and resulting effects should be.

E

Education

Experiences that influence the way people perceive themselves in relation to their social, cultural, and physical environments; a complex and purposeful process for expediting learning.

Educational Assessment

A process whereby health planners seek to assess the causes of a particular health behavior by identifying, sorting, and categorizing three classes of factors that may affect health behavior: predisposing, enabling, and reinforcing factors. An educational assessment examines behavioral and environmental conditions linked to quality-of-life concerns or health status to determine what causes them and identifies factors that can be targeted for change. In health promotion and education planning, the educational assessment is concerned with factors that influence behavior and living conditions of people who are at risk for identified health problems (Green & Kreuter, 1991, 1999). Educational assessment is Phase 4 in the PRECEDE/PROCEED Model. Formerly called *educational diagnosis. See Enabling Factor, PRECEDE/ PROCEED Model, Predisposing Factor,* and *Reinforcing Factor.*

Educational Concept

A summary of the major foci of a particular lesson plan, written in the learner's language; also known as *conceptual learning.* See *Lesson Plan.*

Educational Goal

What an instructor expects to accomplish in an educational session. Setting such goals gives direction to the entire program.

Example: "The participant will recognize behaviors that tend to promote health."

Educational Objective

A specific statement written in one of three domains: cognitive (acquiring knowledge and information intellectually), affective (knowledge coupled with associations such as emotions, values, and attitudes), and psychomotor (inclusion of motor skills and coordination and development of behavioral patterns).

Example: "At the conclusion of this session, the participant will be able to define high blood pressure."

Educational Tools

Leaflets, videotapes, slides, bulletin boards, overhead transparencies, PowerPoint slide presentation material, chalkboards, and other audiovisual support items. Also known as *educational aids* and *educational materials*.

Education Entertainment

A form of health communication in which educational content and information is intentionally incorporated into a less formal program format such as the use of songs, comics, skits, and movies, in an effort to promote health.

Enabling Factor

Any skill, resource, or vehicle created by forces or systems within a society that facilitates the performance of a health action by individuals or organizations, including the availability of and access to health care, personnel, personal health skills, and outreach clinics. Enabling factors also include barriers to action created by societal forces or systems, such as limited access to health care facilities; inadequate resources, income, or health insurance; and restrictive laws, rules, regulations, and policies (Green & Kreuter, 1999).

Entry-Level Health Educator

A person who has obtained the skills, knowledge, and competencies required to perform as a health educator through the successful completion of a bachelor's, master's, or doctoral degree from an accredited college or university, with a major emphasis in health education. There are seven areas of responsibilities and competencies for entry-level health educators, each containing a number of subcompetencies:

1. Assessing individual and community needs for health education
2. Planning effective health education programs
3. Implementing health education programs
4. Evaluating the effectiveness of health education programs
5. Coordinating the provision of health education services
6. Acting as a resource person in health education
7. Communicating health and health education needs, concerns, and resources

Environment

The physical, social, emotional, and spiritual influences on human functioning and behavior, including animate and inanimate surroundings, and the external and internal surroundings that influence health and behavior.

Environmental Assessment

Examination of factors in the social and physical environments to determine whether or not these factors are linked to a person's behavior and identification of any impact the factors may have on behavior change. Factors outside of the individual that have a bearing on health, behavior, and quality of life include lead from paint in older homes, which may cause lead poisoning in children; secondhand smoke inhaled by nonsmokers, such as children in homes of smoking parents or older siblings; and gun violence and homicide (Windsor, Baranowski, Clark, & Cutter, 1994). Also defined as "a systematic assessment of factors in the social and physical environment that interact with behavior to produce health effects or quality-of-life outcomes" (Green & Kreuter, 1999, p. 505). See *Environmental Factors* and *PRECEDE/PROCEED Model*.

Environmental Factors

Specific items or elements determined through environmental diagnosis to be causally linked to health goals or to quality-of-life problems identified through social and epidemiological diagnoses. Also included are factors that are external to individuals or groups but may influence their behavior. See *Environmental Assessment, Epidemiological Assessment,* and *Social Assessment.*

Examples: Housing conditions, air, water, noise, rapid social change, crowding, access to services, light, isolation

Environmental Health

The comprehensive study and management of environmental conditions and principles that influence the health and well-being of individuals, groups, and communities.

Epidemic

The rapid spread of a disease among individuals in a given population clearly in excess of what is normally expected within a geographical area. Epidemics usually affect susceptible members of a population and may last over a certain period of time.

Examples: The AIDS epidemic, affecting all countries; the plague (black death), which struck Europe during the Middle Ages (starting in 1347); excess cases of obesity among a certain population

Epidemiological Assessment

The second phase in the PRECEDE framework concerned with pinpointing important health problems and their causes in a target population. In health education, epidemiological assessment is conducted to determine which interventions may be needed most, based on data gathered from health investigations (Green & Kreuter, 1999). See *Health Indicator* and *PRECEDE/PROCEED Model.*

Epidemiology

The study of disease in terms of distribution, occurrence, determinants, and control in a defined human population.

Ethics

A branch of philosophy focusing on whether a conduct is good or bad or right or wrong. Ethics includes values or standards designed to shed light on the relative rightness or wrongness of actions based on moral principles, professionally endorsed and practiced.

More narrowly, ethics refers to a code or standard established by a profession to govern conduct among members. With reference to health education, the Society for Public Health Education (SOPHE) has adopted a code of ethics for health educators, who need to be aware of the ethical concerns and issues confronting them in the profession.

In 1993, SOPHE published a revised summary code of ethics, noting that "health educators take on profound responsibility in using educational processes to promote health and influence human well-being. Ethical precepts that guide these processes must reflect the right of individuals and communities to make the decisions affecting their lives." AAHE also developed health education ethics, laying out a "common set of values designed to guide health educators in resolving many of the ethical dilemmas experienced in professional life" (1994, p. 197). The code of ethics was further revised in 1999. These guidelines for professional conduct require from health educators a commitment to behave ethically and to encourage and support the ethical behavior of others. (Copies of the latest version of these documents can be obtained from their authors; see Part Two.)

Ethnicity

Identification of individuals or groups with their ancestral origin and their sense of holding shared beliefs, values, norms, and lifestyle.

Etiology

The study of the causes or origins of disease or health problems, taking into account all predisposing factors of the disease.

Evaluation

The comparison of an object of interest against a standard of acceptability. Evaluation can be considered as giving an account or appraisal of what has been done or attaching a value to a program or project. This includes the level or quality of performance, suitability or appropriateness of material used, and budget constraints where applicable (Windsor, Baranowski, Clark, & Cutter, 1994).

In the health education field, evaluation is the act of examining the worth of a program, usually measuring it against a set of predetermined objectives or a standard of acceptability. It involves the process, outcome, and impact of a program or project and demonstrates whether the program reached the desired goals and objectives. The main purpose of evaluation, with specific reference to health education programs, is to improve programs and provide feedback to professionals concerning their strengths and weaknesses, as well as to determine if objectives are being or were met and whether people learned from the programs. See *Formative Evaluation, Impact Evaluation, Outcome Evaluation,* and *Process Evaluation.*

Evaluation Research

Research is intended to produce evidence in support of a testable hypothesis to demonstrate a convincing cause-and-effect relationship between an educational intervention and its outcome. Evaluation research is concerned with the appraisal of the impact of an innovation on individuals or groups. It involves the application of scientific methodologies to test hypotheses concerning the impact or effectiveness of one or more interventions. One of the main objectives of evaluation research is to obtain knowledge that is generalizable in similar groups or populations in other settings (Windsor, Baranowski, Clark, & Cutter, 1994).

Evaluation research has been described as "an evaluation using an experimental or quasi-experimental design conducted to establish the efficacy or effectiveness—internal and/or external validity—and cost effectiveness or cost benefit of an intervention among a defined population at risk for a specific impact or outcome rate during a defined period of time" (Windsor et al., 1994, p. 15).

Evidence-Based Health Education

The practice of selecting from the scientific literature information on programs that have been implemented and have demonstrated evidence of effectiveness in accomplishing the intended outcomes and then using similar strategies to implement and evaluate these programs in different settings.

Excluded Populations

Groups of individuals who may not be typically included in population surveys or research. They may reside in hotels or have other nontraditional living arrangements and therefore may not be tracked.

Exit Interview

A structured interview required by master's students in some schools of public health after they have completed their didactic units and field practica. Students are required to prepare and submit a professional portfolio prior to the interview. Exit interviews are also used with employees who are leaving a company.

External Validity

The degree to which conclusions drawn from research or evaluation are appropriate when applied to other similar settings or populations outside the study. It is the extent to which the program or study can be applied or generalized to other populations with the expectation of producing similar effects. Also known as *generalizability*.

Extrinsic Motivation

Stimulating behavior by the expectation of a reward or avoidance of punishment. Extrinsic motivation is often used to encourage people to participate in a health education program.

Example: Incentives such as lotteries, drawings, raffles, or other financial rewards extrinsically motivate a person to participate in a health education program.

F

Faith-Based Programs

Programs that specifically target churches, temples, mosques, and other places of worship in order to focus on a captive audience and for easy access to families and the communities for health interventions. Initiating health education and promotion programs in places of worship may be more meaningful and personal to some community groups. The belief is that a broader special population can be reached through faith-based initiatives.

Example: The church is a hub of social and educational activities for many African American families; therefore, it is prudent to extend this influence into areas of health where there is a great need for intervention (Lim, Modeste, & Williams, 2003).

Family Planning

A process whereby couples can determine the number of children they would like to have and the spacing of one birth from another, taking into account the health of the mother as well as that of the fetus. Also includes the choice of an appropriate method that will help them realize their goal.

Family Violence

Physical force used against one or more members of a family by another family member with the intent to cause bodily harm, injury, or death.

Examples: The maltreatment of children by parents or other adult family members; physical or sexual abuse by a spouse or intimate partner intended to hurt or cause injury; neglect or abandonment of children by parents; emotional ill-treatment of family members that can affect their health and well-being

Feedback

Verbal or nonverbal responses of a learner that the educator may interpret and use to guide learning, or a two-way communication used to evaluate the effectiveness of communication.

Field Theory

The contention that forces in a group influence one another. The theory holds that behavior results from interactions between forces that pressure a group to move toward a goal and forces working to resist change. These forces tend to work against one another; when the resisting forces outweigh the driving forces, no action is taken because the behavior is blocked (Diamond, 1992). Field theory is important to health educators in that it helps clarify why certain behaviors (health behaviors) are motivated and others are blocked (Butler, 2000).

Example: In a smoking cessation program, knowledge of the health risks involved in smoking and legislation restricting smoking are driving forces for change, but the pleasure one gets from smoking, peer pressure from smoking buddies, and fear of gaining weight after quitting can act as resisting forces. If these resisting forces outweigh the driving forces, the chances for positive behavior change are remote.

Focus Group

A type of qualitative methodology or research technique in which an experienced moderator leads a group of respondents (generally eight to twelve persons) through an informal discussion of a selected problem or issue, allowing group members to talk freely about their thoughts, feelings, opinions, insights, attitudes, misconceptions, and beliefs about the problem. To gather information in health education research, the moderator or interviewer often uses a detailed protocol consisting of open-ended and in-depth questions (Bryant & Gulitz, 1993).

Focus groups are often used in needs assessment to help health educators understand why people think or act in a certain way, and all group members have an equal chance to participate in a discussion (Graeff, Elder, & Mills-Booth, 1993; Soriano, 1995). Focus groups provide an excellent opportunity for observing behavior during a needs assessment. Depending on the topic, participants for a focus group are usually selected on the basis of certain attributes, such as students in a class, parents with disabled children, women who smoke during pregnancy, or low-income families. See *Needs Assessment.*

Force Field Analysis

A graphic examination of a problem based on Lewin's field theory (Baulcomb, 2003), which assumes that any situation is a temporary balance between opposing forces. Driving forces that facilitate change and those that restrain change are identified and rated according to the analyzer's perception.

Formative Evaluation

Evaluation undertaken during the planning and implementation phases of a program, with the intent of using the information gained to determine program effectiveness and to revise and improve the program while it is ongoing. Formative evaluation also provides information on the kinds of outcomes that are needed and how they can be achieved. Investigators look at the immediate or short-term effects of a program in an effort to improve its implementation (Bedworth & Bedworth, 1992; Windsor, Baranowski, Clark, & Cutter, 1994).

Formative Research

Preliminary research conducted prior to the full planning or implementation of a research or program strategy. It may include a pilot study or pilot testing of a questionnaire or survey instrument to determine its acceptability. Also known as *formative evaluation,* especially in evaluations of programs or interventions for their appropriateness and immediate impact. Also defined as "any combination of measurements obtained and judgments made before or during the implementation of materials, methods, activities, or programs to control, assure, or improve the quality of performance or delivery" (Green & Kreuter, 1999, p. 506). See *Pilot Testing*.

Example: Rather than waiting until the end of a smoking cessation program to evaluate its effectiveness, program planners conduct formative evaluation to provide immediate feedback about the quality of the program in order to improve it while the program is ongoing. This evaluation would include information from a variety of sources, including program participants and program providers both before and during program implementation.

G

Gantt Chart

A timetable that shows each activity in a program plan that extends from the beginning to the finish date. A program manager can use this chart at any given time to see the activities that are about to begin, those that are taking place, those that have been completed, and those due to be completed.

Sample Gantt Chart for an Eight-Month Program

Activities	May-June	July-Aug.	Sept.-Oct.	Nov.-Dec.
Do preliminary planning	X			
Conduct needs assessment	X			
Plan program		X		
Contact community		X		
Conduct recruitment and training		X		
Implement program			X	
Evaluate program and follow up				X
Disseminate information				X

Gatekeeper

An intermediary between the sources of a health promotion message and the audience to whom that health message is being directed: community leaders, clergy, parents, school principals, tribal leaders and chiefs, or anyone in control with whom one must work to gain entrance to the audience or the community (Emlet & Hall, 1991; McKenzie, Pinger, & Kotecki, 2002).

Examples: Working with a schoolteacher or principal to gain entrance into the school before implementing a program for schoolchildren; in cultures where husbands are considered gatekeepers, working with husbands prior to implementing family planning education for wives in a community.

General Adaptation Syndrome (GAS)

The body's unsuccessful attempt to adapt to a stressor, resulting in a health deficit.

Generational Epidemic

Any health and other problem passed from parent to offspring.

Examples: Many alcoholics are themselves children of alcoholics; a number of child abusers are victims of child abuse.

Genomics

The branch of science that seeks to provide a clearer understanding of the role genetics play in the etiology or root cause of disease. Genomics helps identify genetic markers and explain the connection between the genes and disease in an effort to prevent disease, as well as to detect certain diseases in their early stage, thus making treatment safer and more effective.

Geographic Information System (GIS)

A system of mapping that uses computers to capture, store, manipulate, integrate, analyze, and display data related to geographical positions or images on a map. Such data are organized for performing statistical analysis by government entities, and environmental management, resource management, engineering, and other businesses. Public health officials use GIS technology to advance information toward more efficient management of the public's health. Information can be gathered, managed, and used for the advancement of health research and program development and implementation, as well as to provide knowledge of where people live geographically and the health-related problems they share, all in an effort to enhance the well-being of populations.

Globalization

The extension of health care and health systems beyond national borders and into world regions to involve new communities and to partner with other institutions in the health field to ensure health protection and wellness for all people.

Global Warming

A gradual increase in the temperature of the earth's surface. Such an increase may cause human health problems and other biological concerns, including an increase in carbon dioxide levels, which may in turn lead to certain alterations in the earth's geographical patterns and climate.

Goal

A statement of broad intent that provides direction in making program decisions; a long-range target toward which behavior change is directed. Goals are used to describe desired levels or resources and expected outcomes, or what should happen as a result of, say, health education programs. Goals are global expectations formulated to include all components of a program.

Examples: "The goal of this program is to develop a child bicycle helmet intervention aimed at reducing head injuries in children." "The goal is to gain an increase in knowledge regarding African American pregnant smokers."

Group Dynamics

The process of interaction between a person and other members of a group; the interaction is concerned with the effect of a group on an individual's readiness to change or maintain, for example, certain health standards or norms.

Group Process

The application of educational and communication principles in group situations in which each member is actively involved in the decision-making process. The group is headed by a leader who determines how the group functions, encourages participation, and prompts for ideas. Group process can facilitate problem solving and decision making through creative thinking to increase credibility and acceptance of recommended health programs and practices.

H

Harm Reduction

Practical strategies as an alternative to total abstinence to teach and encourage people how to reduce the risks of harming themselves. Reducing exposure to health risk behaviors, or practices that may potentially cause physical or psychological harm to the body (Stratton, Shetty, Wallace, & Bondurant, 2001).

Health

The physical, mental, social, and spiritual well-being and fitness that individuals enjoy. Health is not just freedom from disease but is multidimensional and is to a large extent culturally defined.

Health may be defined as the quality of a person's physical, psychological, and sociological functioning in a variety of personal and social situations (Bedworth & Bedworth, 1992). Health is also the ability to survive or adapt to disruptions among the structural, social, and personal components of the individual's health system, as well as to the environment in which the person lives.

Health Advising

"A process of informing and assisting individuals or groups in making decisions and solving problems related to health" (1990 Joint Committee on Health Education Terminology, 1991, p. 105).

Health Advocacy

The employment of specific approaches, processes, guidelines, resources, and strategies to bring about social or organizational change on behalf of a particular interest group or population and to influence public or private policy choices (Carey, Chapman, & Gaffney, 1994; Howze & Redman, 1992; Lupton, 1994).

Advocacy is one of the strategies used by community groups and decision makers to address barriers that impede successful health education intervention. Health advocates can influence governments, organizations, and individuals on health matters.

Example: A group of health professionals takes a position on the issue of cigarette advertising on billboards that target minority communities and initiates actions that could influence the public and policymakers to design laws prohibiting such billboards in those communities.

Labonte (1994) identifies three facets in advocacy in health professional practice. Professionals can offer health-related knowledge and analytical skills to already established community advocacy groups, health institutions can play a role in legitimizing advocacy concerns of community groups by helping to create appropriate policy documents and defining the importance of social life through the services they offer, and health professionals can take a position on public health policy issues at the local, state, or national government levels, including current social welfare reforms, community housing needs, and pertinent environmental standards.

Health Agency

A government or private organization established for the protection and improvement of people's health, such as the World Health Organization (WHO), the National Institutes of Health (NIH), a national ministry of health, county departments of health, the Centers for Disease Control and Prevention (CDC), the National Kidney Foundation, and the Epilepsy Foundation of America.

Health agencies maintain vital health records, monitor disease, and provide direct services and health education to clients through workshops, seminars, and printed materials.

Health Behavior

Behavior directed at promoting, protecting, and maintaining health, as well as reducing disease risks and early death. It includes personal attributes such as beliefs, expectations, values, perceptions, prevention, behavior patterns, actions, and habits that relate to health maintenance, restoration, and improvement. Living conditions, eating habits, exercise habits, and other activities undertaken to prevent disease are also relevant (Bedworth & Bedworth, 1992; Glantz, Lewis, & Rimer, 1990; Green & Kreuter, 1999).

Health Belief Model (HBM)

A theoretical model, first developed by a group of psychologists to help explain why people did or did not use health services, according to which behavior is a function of knowledge, beliefs, and attitudes. It proposes that behaviors related to health can be credited to cognitive decision-making measures and skills (Finfgeld, Wongvatunyu, Conn, Grando, & Russell, 2003; Rosenstock, 1991; Strecher & Rosenstock, 1997).

The model describes and predicts health behavior in terms of beliefs and perceptions about illness, cost of care, and benefits that may accrue. It is frequently used by health educators to predict, describe, and explain health-related behavior based on a person's perceptions and belief patterns. The model is based on the assumption that a person must believe that he or she will develop a health problem in order to take action. The main influences on behavior are perceived susceptibility to a disease, perceived severity of a disease, perceived costs and benefits of taking preventive action, perceived barriers to taking action, and cues to action (advice from peers, mass media campaigns, illness of a family member, or a newspaper article relating to the problem). There must be sufficient concern for health on the individual's part to make health issues relevant.

Health Benefit

A valued improvement or outcome in quality of life that can be attributed to the process of health care.

Example: A person with a heart problem attends a live-in cardiovascular health promotion program involving nutrition, exercise, and other health-related practices and receives the benefit of extending life expectancy without a major heart attack for several years.

Health Care Delivery System

An organized system of services, equipment, personnel, and facilities through which individuals, families, or communities receive health care, including diagnosis, treatment and preventive measures, and patient education for the purpose of promoting, maintaining, and restoring health.

Example: The Loma Linda Centers for Health Promotion and the Kaiser Permanente health care systems include health promotion, education, and preventive services. In these systems, participants are diagnosed, treated, and placed in preventive care and health maintenance programs involving dietary changes, weight loss, smoking cessation, periodic screening, exercise, immunization, and other practices that may help restore or maintain health.

Health Care Provider

Anyone who takes care of a person needing some form of medical or psychological help. Nurses, physicians, dentists, podiatrists, health educators, physical therapists, occupational therapists, psychologists, paramedics, optometrists, practical nurses, nurse practitioners, physician assistants, village health workers, dental hygienists, speech therapists, dietitians, nutritionists, and certain health care corporations are all health care providers.

Health Communication

Informing, influencing, and motivating audiences about important health issues. As defined by the Centers for Disease Control and Prevention, "health communication is the crafting and delivery of messages and strategies, based on consumer research, to promote the health of individuals and communities" (Roper, 1993, p. 179).

Aimed at influencing individual behavior and reducing health risks, health communication involves a series of successive stages, such as examining background information to see what exists in the community, setting communication objectives, analyzing and segmenting target audiences, developing and pretesting messages to be communicated to consumers, selecting channels of communication (see *Communication Channel*), developing a plan for communication activities, implementing the communication strategy, evaluating the effectiveness of the activities, and providing feedback for improvement and more effective planning.

Health Consultant

A technical expert in the field of health education, health promotion, health administration, or health services who has influence in planning and advising on health matters but no direct power to make changes. Health consultants may be called in by private health organizations, schools, colleges, government health departments, and ministries of health in foreign countries to work with committees and health professionals advising on health matters and possible programs or projects to be planned and implemented.

Health Counseling

Interpreting a health problem to learners or others as a means of helping them find a solution. Health counseling may be provided by health educators, nurses, physicians, other health professionals, agencies, or organizations on an individual or group basis, depending on the situation (Bedworth & Bedworth, 1992; Okonski, 2003). Health counseling could be as valuable as conventional clinical activities in preventing disease.

Example: A person who has been diagnosed with hypertension and has a family history of the disease is referred to a health educator or nurse, who explains and interprets what hypertension is all about, the importance of taking action to prevent early disability, the types of foods to include in or delete from the diet, the benefits of exercise, and sources for additional help. Counseling by health professionals is effective in helping people change dietary, smoking, and other behaviors that negatively affect health.

Health-Directed Behavior

Actions deliberately aimed at protecting or improving one's health; also known as *health behavior*. See *Health Behavior*.

Examples: Adopting a low-fat or low-salt diet or a diet containing less meat; the decision to assign a sober driver if the designated driver was drinking alcohol; wearing bicycle helmets and seat belts

Health Disparities

Differences in health care experienced by certain segments of the population, often as a consequence of unequal access to care. The National Institutes of Health (2003) define health disparities as "differences in the incidence, prevalence, mortality, and burden of diseases and other adverse health conditions that exist among specific population groups in the United States."

Health Education

An educational process concerned with providing a combination of approaches to lifestyle change that can assist individuals, families, and communities in making informed decisions on matters that affect the restoration, achievement, and maintenance of health. Health education is also a deliberately structured discipline or profession that provides learning opportunities about health through interactions between educators and learners using a variety of learning experiences. This process of learning can enable people to voluntarily change conditions or modify behavior for health enhancement. See *Behavior Modification* and *Health Enhancement.*

Health education is much more than factual information. It includes all those experiences and skills that affect the way people think and feel about their health, and it motivates them to put information into practice (Bedworth & Bedworth, 1992; Greenberg, 1992; McKenzie, Pinger, & Kotecki, 2002).

Health Education Administrator

A person trained in health, health education, education, and administration who combines these skills in organizing, administering, supervising, and evaluating health education programs.

Health education administrators are concerned with providing direction and leadership to health agencies (voluntary or governmental) or schools and seeing that program goals are achieved. They also organize health education programs on the district, community, and state levels.

Health education administrators should have training and experience in health administration and health education, in relationship to the health care system, and they must be able to use effective communication. For role delineation, functions, and responsibilities, see Bedworth and Bedworth (1992, chap. 10).

Examples: A health education administrator may function in a health department, hospital, or HMO as head of the health education department. A school health education administrator serves at the city, county, or state level.

Health Education Competency

The achievement of skills needed by health educators to perform successfully in a variety of settings in the workplace. Competency-based preparation in health education skills and responsibilities as established by the National Commission for Health Education Credentialing.

Health Education Coordinator

"A professional health educator who is responsible for the management and coordination of all health education policies, activities, and resources within a particular setting or circumstance" (1990 Joint Committee on Health Education Terminology, 1991, p. 104).

Health Education Curriculum Guide

A tool used to plan courses to encourage positive health attitudes and behavior in students, helping them understand health problems and issues and integrate concepts associated with physical, mental, social, spiritual, and emotional well-being. The curriculum guide is designed to include such items as family living, drugs, growth and development, nutrition, safety, environment, community health, and mental health and should be flexible to allow for adaptation in individual school districts.

Health Education Diagnosis

The identification and delineation of factors that predispose, enable, or reinforce a specific health behavior in a person or population. It is also referred to as *educational assessment* in the PRECEDE/PROCEED Model. See *Educational Assessment* and *PRECEDE/PROCEED Model.*

Health Education Field

The multidisciplinary practice concerned with planning, implementing, and evaluating health education programs that are intended to empower individuals, families, communities, and community organizations to achieve, protect, and sustain health on the personal, environmental, and social levels.

Health Education Policy

A plan of action focused on fostering the development of health promotion programs, including the training and utilization of health education personnel.

With the increased use of health education in treatment and illness prevention, as well as the focus on personal health behaviors and practice, health educators are involved in policymaking pertinent to specific programs or projects.

Health Education Practice

The application of knowledge and skills based on educational theories to promote health and lifestyle changes in a target population. See *Health Education.*

Examples: Conducting a weight loss program, an antidrug campaign, or a harm reduction education program; teaching cancer prevention education to high-risk groups

Health Education Process

The continuum or series of learning experiences that enable people to make decisions, modify behaviors, and change social and environmental conditions to be more conducive to health enhancement.

Example: Providing opportunities for pregnant teenagers to receive prenatal education and promoting breast-feeding

Health Education Program

A combination of activities based on needs assessment, broad principles of education, and evaluation targeted at a specific population and usually involving the setting of goals and objectives.

Health Education Standards

A framework indicating what students in the health education profession should know and be able to do. Knowledge and skills essential to the development of health literacy include the ways of communicating, reasoning, and investigating that characterize health education. Health education standards are *not* merely facts. Rather, they identify the knowledge and skills students should master in order to attain a high level of competency in health education. Skills may include problem solving, decision making, goal setting, critical thinking, interpersonal communication, media, health literacy, advocacy, mathematical skills, and the ability to collaborate and apply knowledge from multiple content areas in a work setting. The ultimate goal of health education standards is health enhancement and improved personal, family, and community health. (A booklet containing the official health education standards of the American Association for Health Education is available; see Part Two.)

Health Education Tool

Any material or teaching aid, such as a film, video, set of slides or overhead transparencies, or pamphlet, designed to improve the learning process in health education. Such tools also include advertisements on television and radio. See *Educational Tools*.

Health Educator

An individual who specializes in health education through academic preparation and serves in such roles as program planning, intervention, advocacy, and policy development to help individuals make informed decisions in matters affecting their health.

"A health educator is a highly trained individual who attempts to improve the health of people through use of the educational process" (Bedworth & Bedworth, 1992, p. 447). A health educator may have specialized interests such as community health, school health, patient education, or cooperative or worksite health education.

A health educator is "a professionally prepared individual who serves in a variety of roles and is specifically trained to use appropriate educational strategies and methods to facilitate the development of policies, procedures, interventions, and systems conducive to the health of individuals, groups, and communities" (2000 Joint Committee on Health Education Terminology, 2001, p. 6).

A health educator may function in a variety of settings, such as community health agencies, public health agencies, worksites, schools, colleges, universities, hospitals, clinics, voluntary health organizations, health maintenance organizations, professional organizations, and other organizations and agencies with a health education emphasis or program. Persons from diverse backgrounds, such as nurses, physicians, social workers, and educators, may also become health educators and function within the field or include health promotion and education as a component of their work.

Health Enhancement

A dimension of health promotion pertaining to the aim of reaching higher levels of wellness beyond the mere absence of disease and infirmity. Health enhancement begins with people who are basically healthy, but it is not limited to the well population. Persons with chronic diseases such as cardiovascular problems may be provided with exercise facilities and encouraged to exercise regularly in order to improve their level of wellness (Chenoweth, 1991).

Health Equity

The concept that everyone should have a fair and impartial opportunity to achieve full health potential and that equal opportunities for health should

Dictionary of Public Health Promotion and Education

be created to lower health differentials among individuals or groups. Unfortunately, this concept of fair and equal opportunity in health care for everyone has not been achieved in the United States, as it has in some other countries, and does not presently seem likely, given current problems of access to health care, available resources, and ethnic concerns. See *Access to Health Care.*

Health Facility

Any setting, such as a building, health education center, health clinic, hospital, nursing home, sports medicine clinic, or weight loss clinic, where health care is provided and health resources are available.

Health Fair

A community health promotion program set up in a mall, hall, or other place frequented by consumers. Health fairs are also conducted at worksites for employees and their families. Booths are used to demonstrate information on cholesterol, hypertension, diabetes, dental screening and care, weight control, and nutrition in relation to specific conditions and diseases. Videos, films, audiovisual displays, exhibits, pamphlets, handouts, and other health-related materials can help raise the level of consciousness about health issues among members of the community. Other areas of health interest may be included as appropriate to the specific community.

Participants in a health fair may be drawn from community groups, including the county health department, churches, schools, worksites, hospitals, fire and police departments, medical and dental auxiliaries, health agencies, and associations such as the American Cancer Society, the American Heart Association, and the American Lung Association (Breckon, Harvey, & Lancaster, 1994).

Healthful School Environment

A school environment offering safe and clean school buildings and grounds (including parking lots, swimming pools, playgrounds, rest rooms, locker rooms, and science laboratories); clean food preparation and serving areas;

adequate classroom lighting, ventilation, and noise control; and protection against radiation, asbestos, and lead. In addition, safety requires adequate disposal of toxic and other waste material, smoke-free classrooms, drug-free school grounds, and avoidance of crime and violence. The health environment forms the basis for other health services development.

Health Indicator

A marker of a health problem, such as mortality (e.g., number of female deaths from all causes per 100,000 population), morbidity (e.g., number of people with a chronic disease such as diabetes or number of children under ten years of age with anemia), disability (e.g., number of persons incapacitated or disadvantaged sufficiently to warrant special care), or nutritional status, that gives clues to life expectancy. Health indicators are indispensable to health agencies, health departments, and countries attempting to control disease and to health educators and health care workers for planning health education and public health activities. See *Morbidity* and *Mortality*.

Health Informatics

The use of information theories, logic, algorithms, computers, and other information technologies to improve the health of individuals, groups, communities, and nations. "The systematic application of information and technology to research, theory, practice, and learning applied to health" (2000 Joint Committee on Health Education Terminology, 2001, p. 7).

Health Information

The content of communications based on credible, systematic, and scientific data and methodologies as they relate to health issues, policies, programs, services, and other aspects of individual and public health that affect individuals and communities.

Health Information System

A data collection scheme to provide information about the impact of a health education program and the effect it is having on its target group or community. Data collected are saved for retrieval as needed for research, teaching, statistical information, and program evaluation.

Example: A county health agency can retrieve data from a health information system to help with assessing community needs and identifying specific effects of past projects.

Health Intervention

Any health-related measure taken to improve the health of an individual or a community; this may involve diagnosing, preventing, treating, and managing disease conditions, injury, or disability.

Health Investigation

Collecting and evaluating health-related information from community members and using this information to describe the occurrence of a disease, its possible causes and symptoms, and its association with other factors and environmental exposure to substances that might be related to the disease.

Health Literacy

The ability to understand and navigate health information necessary to access health care, increase health knowledge, and identify factors that affect the health of individuals and communities. It includes the ability to read and follow health instructions, including prescriptions; to obtain and interpret essential health information; and to adopt health-promoting behaviors.

Health Locus of Control

People's attribution of responsibility for their own health, reflecting whether they believe that their health is controlled by factors relating to their own behaviors or by external factors over which they have no control. See *Locus of Control.*

Health Maintenance Organization (HMO)

An organized prepaid comprehensive health care delivery system, public or private, set up to provide health care maintenance and treatment services in a geographical area. The idea originated in the late 1940s with the Kaiser Foundation health plan. Payment to an HMO is usually through a reimbursement plan of predetermined periodic prepayments made by or on behalf of participating individuals.

HMOs focus on reducing health care costs and incorporating health education, health promotion, and disease prevention as integral parts of the medical system. HMOs may contract with independent physicians or employ physicians in various specialties. The physicians may be paid a salary or a flat fee for each patient per month. Typically, an employer pays a fixed fee in return for all necessary health care for employees, who may or may not be required to make a copayment.

Health Outcome

A specified measurable change, positive or negative, in an individual, patient, or population that results from health promotion or health care. It includes results from the impact of a program on participants and an examination of whether new behavior is associated with improved health or whether changes in behavior led to health status outcomes. See *Impact Evaluation.*

Example: Health educators conduct a needs assessment to determine what programs ought to be offered in a community and as a result select a prenatal education program for teenage mothers. Health outcomes resulting from this program may include lower medical costs, fewer babies with low birth weight, fewer pregnancy complications, fewer cesarean sections, and shorter hospital stays.

Health Outcome Evaluation

An evaluation "designed to assess intervention efficacy or effectiveness in producing long-term changes (e.g., 1–10 years) in the incidence or prevalence of morbidity rates, mortality rates, or other health status indicators for a clinically diagnosed medical condition among a defined population at risk" (Windsor, Baranowski, Clark, & Cutter, 1994, p. 14).

Health Parity

The provision of an adequate level of health care that is culturally based, comprehensive, appropriate, community-centered, and sustainable. The health services are designed for further prevention and quality of life for all members of the community and address issues such as housing and sanitation, employment and income inequalities, educational opportunities, environmental health concerns, and social and economic justice. See *Health Equity.*

Health Personnel

Persons who provide health care services either as members of institutions or as individual practitioners. These may include such professionals as health educators, nurses, nurse practitioners, physicians, dentists, pharmacists, and physician assistants.

Health Policy

A health-directed plan of action designed to influence the delivery of health care services, often consisting of written guidelines to help regulate health care, health services, and health programs. The health policy process involves input from federal, state, and local governments, legislative and executive bodies, advocacy groups, corporations, independent agencies, insurers, health care providers, the media, and educational institutions.

Health policy involves being employed in decision making on several health promotion and education issues, and many health behavior problems have serious implications for policy. Health policy formation and implementation interrelate with the behaviors, attitudes, and knowledge of the public in matters affecting health.

Health educators need an adequate understanding of the development of policy and should participate in policymaking whenever opportunities arise. Health educators are valuable resource persons in the course of health policy formation. Some examples of health policies include bicycle helmet use policies, seat belt policies, and policies for smoke-free schools and workplaces.

Health Problem

Any condition of being unsound in body, mind, or spirit that adversely affects one's quality of life.

Health-Promoting Environment

An environment in which people can breathe clean air, drink and use clean water, and have adequate sewage disposal systems so as to reduce disease and disability and in which health and safety policies and legislation are in place to protect employees, staff, patients, clients, and everyone else in that environment.

Health-Promoting Schools

Schools that provide and encourage a healthy physical environment in which students study, learn, play, and spend most of their day and in which health and health education are part of the curriculum. Health services are also available, and the teachers and staff are included in activities that promote and sustain health.

Health Promotion

The use of a combination of health education and specific interventions, such as antismoking campaigns, breast health month, and diabetes awareness, at the primary level of prevention designed to facilitate behavioral and environmental changes conducive to health enhancement and harm reduction.

Health promotion aims at helping people change to more healthy lifestyles through public participation in various efforts to enhance awareness and create environments that support positive health practices that may result in reducing health risks in a population (Bunton & Macdonald, 1992; Green & Kreuter, 1999).

Health promotion can occur in various settings, such as the community as a whole, hospitals, clinics, churches, organizations such as the YMCA and YWCA, community wellness centers, schools, and worksites.

Tasks include needs assessment, problem identification, development of appropriate goals and objectives, creation of interventions, implementation of interventions, and the evaluation of outcomes or results. Benefits of health promotion information may include changes in attitudes, increased awareness and knowledge, lowered risk for certain health problems, better health status, and improved quality of life.

Professionals who engage in health promotion may include health educators, nurses, physicians, physical therapists, dentists, dental hygienists, social workers, teachers, and nutritionists.

Health Promotion Program

Any program, such as alcohol awareness month, cancer prevention week, obesity reduction seminar, or dental health week, aimed at improving health through behavior and lifestyle changes.

Health Protection

The implementation of strategies that focus on environmental rather than behavioral determinants of health. Emphasis is therefore on providing a wholesome environment in the hope of protecting the health of individuals and communities. Specific areas targeted in today's society may include environmental hazards such as toxic waste sites, industrial chemicals, and exposure to lead, air pollutants, and radon; food and drug safety, with special attention to pesticide residues and microbial contamination; occupational health and safety, such as wearing protective clothing, goggles, and gloves when working with dangerous chemicals; and monitoring workplaces for emerging hazards.

Health Risk Appraisal

Determining the health risks of individuals and needs of targeted populations through the use of special computer software programs. These instruments ask people to respond to a number of questions about their health behavior and health history and may include details such as height, weight, blood pressure, and cholesterol measurements. The information is usually entered into a computer program designed to provide both individual and group results. Results from appraisals may be used to suggest risk reduction activities—reducing weight to normal range, stopping smoking, decreasing consumption of high-fat and high-cholesterol foods, and increased exercise.

Health Status

The measured state of health of an individual or a population, determined by comparison to standardized data. The health status of a population can be measured by birthrates, life expectancy, risk factors, quality-of-life indicators, disease morbidity, access to health care, death rates, and other factors affecting health. An individual's health status can be measured by weight, height, blood pressure, heart rate, family health history, and lifestyle practices regarding smoking and exercise. In measuring the health status of a population, one may want to look beyond these measurements to data and trends about disease, including incidence and prevalence rates, mortality and morbidity data, and environmental factors that may enhance or adversely affect health.

Healthy Community

A community that continuously improves its physical and social environments and expands its resources to enable its citizens to lead healthier lives and support one another in developing their full potential.

Healthy Lifestyle

Patterns of behavior that improve or enhance an individual's quality of life by reducing harm and decreasing susceptibility to poor health outcomes, including behaviors that are shaped from personal values, beliefs, and attitudes, as well as outside forces from one's family, culture, and society.

Healthy People 2010

A nationwide health promotion and disease prevention agenda that sets goals and objectives and is intended to serve as a guide for improving the health of all people living in the United States by the year 2010. The initiative builds on the previous national health promotion and disease prevention objectives, known as Healthy People 2000, and is committed to promoting health and preventing illness, disability, and premature death. Two broad goals are to "increase quality and years of healthy life" and "eliminate health disparities." For more information about Healthy People 2010, go to http://www.health.gov/healthypeople.

Hierarchy of Learning

The three levels of progressive learning:

1. The acquisition of health *facts,* which may include knowledge about certain health issues or the cause and prevention of certain health problems
2. The development of health *attitudes,* or feelings about a health problem
3. The development of *values* that may lead to behavior change

Health educators are well aware that the acquisition of knowledge (health facts) does not necessarily ensure proper health behavior. Health educators must concern themselves with learning situations such as attitudes, beliefs, and values in addition to knowledge (Bedworth & Bedworth, 1992; Shapiro, 1999).

Hierarchy of Needs

A concept developed in the 1950s by Abraham Maslow, who arranged needs in an order of importance from the most basic biological needs to psychological needs concerned with self-actualization, on the assumption that needs lower down in the hierarchy must be met before the motivation to meet higher needs manifests (Benson & Dundis, 2003; Lester, 1990).

There are five basic needs, arranged from lowest to highest hierarchically:

1. Physiological—the need for such basics as food, water, and oxygen
2. Safety—the need for protection
3. Love—the need for a feeling of belonging
4. Esteem—the need to feel appreciated
5. Self-actualization—the need to achieve one's full potential in terms of growth, development, and functioning

The concept is important to health educators, especially those involved in counseling, who must often address issues of self-esteem, safety, and self-actualization (Bedworth & Bedworth, 1992).

Host

Any person or animal that harbors a disease or condition. A squirrel may carry rabies, or cattle may act as host for certain tick-borne diseases. A host may be identified in different ways: A host in which the parasite attains maturity or passes its sexual stage is considered *primary;* a host in which a parasite is in a larval or asexual state is referred to as *intermediate* or *secondary;* and a host in which the organism remains alive but does not undergo development is a *transport* host. See *Carrier.*

Hypothesis

A supposition or a prediction that an investigator makes and sets out to prove. A tentative statement postulating that a relationship exists between two or more variables or characteristics (Creswell, 1994), such as smoking (exposure to tar and other chemicals in cigarettes) and lung cancer (a disease).

A hypothesis may be expressed in the *null* form (e.g., "There is no relationship between hormone therapy and breast cancer in menopausal women") or in the *alternative* form (e.g., "The more that menopausal women use hormone therapy, the more likely it is that they will develop breast cancer").

In scientific research and evaluation, a hypothesis is a prediction of the results of an experiment or study, a tentative proposition to be confirmed or rejected by research (Powers & Knapp, 1990).

Example: On the issue of AIDS and teenagers, a hypothesis statement could be "There is no relationship between teenagers' perception of the risk of AIDS and their intended sexual behavior." This hypothesis could be tested by collecting data or facts from teenagers regarding their perception of the risk for getting AIDS and their behavior intention. These facts will lead to the acceptance or rejection of the hypothesis.

I

Illness Behavior

Activities undertaken by persons in response to their beliefs about being ill to discover what is wrong and what can be done about it. The behavior may be different from what medical assessment finds to be the problem. *Illness* refers to what the person feels is wrong and not what a doctor says or discovers is amiss (Bond & Clark, 2002; Crane & Martin, 2002). See *Health Behavior.*

Example: A person who feels ill may visit a health screening and consultation program where height, weight, and blood pressure measurements are taken and blood tests and possibly an electrocardiogram are performed to discover why she feels ill and to help plan a course of action.

Impact Evaluation

An assessment of the immediate, short-term, and long-term results or effects that a program or some aspect of a program had on the target behaviors (Green & Kreuter, 1999; Windsor, Baranowski, Clark, & Cutter, 1994). Impact evaluation is one of the most comprehensive forms of evaluation and is designed to determine whether a project's objectives have been achieved and whether changes that were observed in the population can be attributed to effects generated by the program. These changes may include predisposing, enabling, and reinforcing factors. See *Enabling Factor, Environmental Factors, Outcome Evaluation, Predisposing Factor, Program Evaluation,* and *Reinforcing Factor.*

Example: A number of people began using condoms after the first session of a promotion program. Impact evaluation looks at the program objectives for immediate changes in predisposing, enabling, reinforcing, behavioral, and environmental factors as well as for long-range changes in morbidity, mortality, and maintenance of a desired behavior (Green & Kreuter, 1999; Windsor et al., 1994).

Incentive

A commodity or condition capable of stimulating action to satisfy a drive or achieve a goal. An incentive is often used as an extrinsic motivational device that may take the form of reward or punishment.

An incentive is something that an individual looks forward to upon completion of a task—a reward. An incentive that is perceived as positive is usually more desirable and effective than one perceived as negative.

Incentives are important in motivating behavior and hence health behavior, but only to the extent that they relate to previous similar behavior. If the incentive used is unfamiliar to the individual, it may have no effect.

Examples: A person may be offered free exercise equipment as a reward for completing a six-week intensive course of exercise and physical fitness or a trip to the Bahamas for losing twenty pounds.

Incidence

A measure of new cases of a disease or the frequency of occurrence of a disease based on new cases in a population within a certain time period. It is the number of instances of persons falling ill during a given time in a specified population.

Incidence rate is often used to indicate the rate at which new events (cases) occur in a population or an estimate of the probability (risk) of people's developing a disease during a specified period of time. In public health, incidence is used as a measurement of morbidity or to express morbidity and is calculated by dividing the number of new cases over a specified period of time by the population at risk and presented as follows:

$$\text{Incidence rate per 1,000} = \frac{\text{Number of new cases of a disease occurring in the population during a specified period of time}}{\text{Number of persons exposed to the risk of developing the disease during that period of time}} \times 1,000$$

Health educators and public health workers need to be aware of the incidence or occurrence of disease in a population to plan appropriate and effective interventions.

Independent Variable

In an experiment, the presumed cause of a phenomenon that can be used to predict the value of another variable in the experiment. An independent variable causes a change in something. The researcher manipulates the independent variable in order to observe its effects on the dependent variable. The independent variable is also referred to as the *predictor variable* in epidemiological research (Powers & Knapp, 1990; Vogt, 1993). See *Dependent Variable*.

Example: To clarify the relationship between obesity and heart disease, weight reduction must also be considered. Participation in a weight reduction program or weight loss (independent variable) may reduce heart disease (dependent variable) in specific individuals.

Inductive Learning

A methodology of learning from examples. It begins with a question such as "What factors predispose a person to developing prostate cancer?" or a hypothesis statement such as "There is no relationship between cigarette smoking and prostate cancer." This is followed by the accumulation of empirical evidence or discoveries, from which conclusions are drawn.

In relation to health education, inductive learning methodology begins with a health problem or issue, followed by an accumulation of empirical evidence, from which conclusions, facts, and answers are drawn or learned. This method of learning is the opposite of deductive learning. See *Deductive Learning*.

Information Overload

A condition that occurs when people have so much information available to them that it is difficult to use the information appropriately or to determine which pieces of information to discard and which to use.

Information Theory

The study of communication systems and the principles governing understanding, control, and predictability in communication. It explains the transmission of information from a source to a final destination.

The message (what is being communicated) begins from the source, which can have a variety of origins (physical environment, learning resources, the health educator, or the individual's own thought processes); is transmitted in words or visual form; is picked up by a communication channel such as radio, television, or newspaper; reaches the receiver; and is then interpreted and used. For a clearer understanding and application of the theory to health education, see Bedworth and Bedworth (1992, pp. 382–384).

Informed Consent

A legal tenet that holds providers responsible for ensuring that consumers or patients understand the risks and benefits associated with a procedure before it is administered.

Research participants must also be made aware of the nature of the research, its benefits, its risks, and the confidentiality of the data to be collected, before deciding whether or not to participate. Informed consent rules are intended to protect subjects, or participants, of research. For ethical and moral reasons, health educators need to obtain informed consent from subjects when carrying out research that involves humans.

Informed consent procedures are usually reviewed by institutional review boards, which exist in major educational institutions, hospitals, and research institutions. A consent form created by the researcher must generally be read and signed by each prospective research participant (Powers & Knapp, 1990).

Injury Prevention

Efforts to reduce the risk of injuries before they happen. Passive approaches to injury prevention include childproof caps on medicine bottles and air bags and automatic seat belt restraints in automobiles. Active behavioral approaches include promoting seat belt and bicycle helmet use.

Dictionary of Public Health Promotion and Education

Innovation-Diffusion Theory

A theory that attempts to identify the process by which an innovation (new program) spreads through society. This theory is useful to health promotion because different social groups may comprehend things differently. Different people identify with and accept innovations differently, which plays an important role in the implementation and success of a program.

Innovation-diffusion theory helps explain how innovations spread from one person to another, one group to another, or throughout a population and how innovations are adopted. The theory describes patterns that target populations follow in adopting a program (Bunton & Macdonald, 1992; McKenzie & Jurs, 1993).

Innovators

The first persons to adopt a new idea or practice after receiving information about it.

In-Service Training

Educational programs for advanced training or review training for persons in professions and on the job.

Example: A workshop for health educators on the job can inform or educate them on a current issue pertinent to their job of which they may be unaware.

Instructional Aids

Written or audiovisual materials used to implement a lesson plan or health promotion presentation.

Internality-Externality Hypothesis of Obesity

A psychological theory proposing that obese people are more responsive to external cues, such as the presence of food or time of day, whereas nonobese people use more internal cues, such as hunger, to guide eating. According to this theory, obese people confronted with an array of palatable-looking foods respond more readily to partaking of these foods and eat more than the nonobese, especially if the food is tasty and tempting. This responsiveness, however, may be related to habits of dieting that obese people develop, either continual on-and-off dieting or refraining entirely from dieting.

Internal Validity

The degree to which an investigator's conclusions correctly describe what actually happened in a study; "the degree to which an observed change in an impact (behavior) or outcome (health status) rate (A) among individuals at risk (B) can be attributed to an intervention (C): Did C cause A to change among B?" (Windsor, Baranowski, Clark, & Cutter, 1994, pp. 14–15). The degree of certainty that a program caused the change that is being measured or the results of an evaluation is the program's internal validity. A study is said to have internal validity when the variables are logically consistent and represent a testable "causal relationship" (Vogt, 1993). See *Validity*.

Intervention

A planned and systematically applied program designed to produce behavior changes or improve health status among individuals or a population at risk. To carry out an intervention, health educators develop instruments such as questionnaires or review existing instruments for readability, ease of comprehension, sensitivity, and validity. This is done prior to the actual implementation of a program and forms part of the basis for program design. Types of interventions may include smoking cessation, exercise classes, and breast self-examination.

Intervention Strategy

A set of programs or policies implemented primarily to have an impact on a specific illness or disease.

Example: A bicycle helmet law mandating that children wear helmets while riding to prevent serious injury and reduce deaths from head injuries

Intrinsic Motivation

Engaging in an action or behavior for its own sake or reward; often contrasted with *extrinsic motivation*. See *Extrinsic Motivation*.

Example: People who exercise because they enjoy the activity in and of itself (intrinsic motivation) are more likely to continue to exercise than people who exercise because they expect to be rewarded (extrinsic motivation).

L

Late Majority

Part of a population or community that is hard to reach or to convince to adopt new information, ideas, or health practices or may be the last to be reached because of difficulty accessing the information, inability to reach the source, or due to cultural, language, or financial barriers.

Leadership

In public health, the process of intentionally influencing others to work toward the goals and objectives of the organization, group, or program.

Learner-Centered Guide

A written document that describes what learners will be doing to achieve their objectives.

Learner Objectives

Brief, clear written statements that describe instructional intent in terms of the desired learning outcomes in three domains: cognitive (knowledge, comprehension), affective (emotional concepts such as interests and attitudes), and psychomotor (motor skills). Learner objectives are stated for individuals and begin with an action verb that is measurable. Also known as *instructional objectives* or *educational objectives*. See *Affective Domain, Educational Objective,* and *Psychomotor Domain.*

Example: "At the end of this session, the student will be able to state the key determinants of health behavior change."

Learning Community

People, including faculty and students working, or interacting together in an integrative learning environment with a structured curriculum of coursework, designed to provide more opportunities for learning to take place more effectively.

Lesson Plan

A document delineating an active educational process in which a learner participates to reach educational goals. An organizational structure for teaching that is built around the ordering of concepts, objectives, learning opportunities, and evaluation procedures within a specific lesson. Also called an *instructional guide.*

Life Events

Significant social changes experienced by individuals as part of everyday life that may have some positive or negative outcomes in the promotion and protection of their health.

Life Expectancy

"The average number of years a person, from a specific cohort, is projected to live from a given point in time" (McKenzie, Pinger, & Kotecki, 2002, p. 69). Life expectancy is one indicator of the health status of a society or a population.

Lifestyle

A complex of related practices or constrained patterns of daily living maintained with some consistency in a person or group. Lifestyle involves cultural, physical, social, mental, spiritual, and environmental actions or characteristics of an individual or group (Grover, Gray, Joseph, Abrahamowicz, & Coupal, 1994; Moorhead, 1992; Sinha, 1992).

Lifestyle is "the culturally, socially, economically, and environmentally conditioned complex of actions characteristic of an individual, group, or community as a pattern of habituated behavior over time that is health related but not necessarily health directed" (Green & Kreuter, 1999, p. 507).

Lifestyle is a determining factor in the state of one's health, because the type of lifestyle one chooses may result in a loss of health or premature death. Lifestyle choices that put people at risk include cigarette smoking, substance use and abuse (including alcohol and other drugs), poor nutritional habits, obesity, and a lack of exercise (Backett, Davison, & Mullen, 1994; Knutsen, 1994; Ornish et al., 1990).

Health education and promotion programs aim at changing lifestyles and behaviors that may put people at risk. However, health educators must keep in mind that individuals retain the right to make their own decisions regarding lifestyle choices.

Lifestyle Diseases

Chronic illnesses that are partly a result of lifestyle choices that are not considered healthy. Choices such as cigarette smoking, drug use, a sedentary life with little or no exercise, poor food selections, and other behavioral factors that can lead to negative health effects.

Lifestyle Habits

Habits that people adopt and practice in their daily lives that have positive or negative effects on their health. Habits promoting positive effects include wearing safety helmets and seat belts; avoiding smoking and secondhand smoke, and other harmful drugs; choosing and eating a nutritious balanced diet that includes whole grains, nuts, fruits, and vegetables; getting adequate hours of sound sleep nightly and sufficient daily exercise; and employing healthy sexual practices. Habits promoting negative effects include refusing to wear seat belts or safety helmets, smoking, taking drugs, making poor nutrition choices, getting insufficient sleep, not exercising, and engaging in unhealthy sexual practices.

Locus of Control

One's perceived source of control over one's environment. Health locus of control posits that health outcomes are determined either by an individual's actions or by external forces beyond one's control. Individuals with an internal locus of control believe that positive or negative events are under their personal control, whereas those with external control beliefs think that important outcomes are the result of luck, chance, or powerful others (Anderson, De Vellis, Sharpe, & Marcoux, 1994; Goodman, Cooley, Sewell, & Leavitt, 1994; Rotter, 1992). Persons with an internal locus of control are more likely to believe that they can influence health outcomes than those with an external locus of control. See *Health Locus of Control*.

Longitudinal Study

A research design in which the same individuals or groups are observed at different points in time over a designated period. A longitudinal study may involve a single cohort with similar characteristics, such as residency in a given geographical area and a specified age range, race or ethnicity, marital status, and socioeconomic status, followed over time to investigate developments with respect to variables being tested.

Example: A group of children born in homes built within half a mile of a toxic waste site may be examined at several points in time over a fifteen- to twenty-year period for the development of certain cancers.

M

Managed Care

A health plan that combines both the financing and the delivery of comprehensive health care services to people who are covered by specific insurance arrangements with health care providers. It is touted as a way of controlling health care costs by encouraging shorter hospital stays or inpatient services, infrequent use of specialists, inclusion of preventive services, and greater management control over both health providers and consumers.

Marketing

"Determination of what programs are wanted or needed by target groups, determination of what the attributes of these programs are, and promotion of such programs" (Breckon, 1997, p. 313). In health care, the promotion of health care services to consumers of such services.

Media Advocacy

"Bringing about policy changes by using the media to put pressure on policy makers. This is accomplished by placing issues on the media agenda through media relations efforts and/or paid advertising, or seeing that issues already on the media agenda are framed from a policy perspective" (Siegel & Doner, 1998, p. 507).

Mentor

An experienced health professional willing to coach a newly employed health care professional on details of the public health arena and the organizations' philosophies and to guide the advancement of the newcomer's career. A mentor may also work with public health students to help develop their leadership skills and career path. From an organizational standpoint, creating an opportunity for employees to be mentored is a key factor in employee satisfaction and organizational success.

Method

In the health education field, a procedure used to determine what communication techniques and strategies should be employed to assist in the learning process. Methods include the use of media and different styles of teaching and learning, such as role-playing, group instruction, class presentations, storytelling, and group discussions. Methods are systematic plans for implementing a program or project. The term *method* is used interchangeably with *methodology.*

In research, the term is used to describe techniques, strategies, and other procedures. The methods or methodology section of the research design gives detailed information on the subject selection, instrumentation, whether a structured questionnaire was developed and pretested, questionnaire content, data collection procedures, and statistical analysis.

Middle Majority

"The segment of the population who adopt a new idea or practice after the innovators or early adopters but before the late adopters, usually influenced by a combination of mass media, interpersonal communications, and endorsement by famous personalities or organizations of which they are members" (Green & Kreuter, 1999, p. 507).

Mission Statement

"A carefully formulated statement that defines the purpose of an organization. It may be a sentence or two in length or several pages. It is the beginning point for most planning procedures" (Breckon, 1997, p. 314).

Example: "The mission of local health departments is to protect, promote, and maintain the health of the entire population of their jurisdiction" (Scutchfield & Keck, 2003, p. 123).

Model

A conceptual basis for how a program or evaluation is supposed to work. A model is usually expressed graphically rather than textually but may be in narrative form, explaining key factors and variables (Cresswell, 1994). A model "serves to objectify and present a certain perspective or point of view about its nature and/or function" (Powers & Knapp, 1990, p. 88).

In public health, health promotion, and health education, a model may be necessary for several reasons, such as helping to explain how behavior occurs, how health education is conducted, and how health education affects ongoing behavior. Programs and evaluations can be based on models, or theories, of human behavior (Windsor, Baranowski, Clark, & Cutter, 1994).

Examples: Two frequently used models in health education are the Health Belief Model and the PRECEDE/PROCEED Model.

Modeling

A person's inclination to imitate another person's behavior. It is learning that takes place through observation of others and is an important process through which socialization occurs. Learning that takes place through modeling is more than just mimicking a behavior and is very influential in the formation of habits and behavior. Modeling begins in early infancy and continues through adulthood; however, the strongest effects are during the early years of life. The effects of modeling can be both good and bad, depending on what is being modeled, and can play an important role in the promotion of healthful practices regarding alcohol, smoking, diet, and exercise.

Examples: Much of the violence seen on television may be modeled by teenagers, who have been influenced since early childhood through television viewing of violent scenes. A child from a home in which both parents never smoked is more likely to model that behavior and never take up smoking during his or her lifetime.

Modifiable Risk Factors

Factors that contribute to the development of chronic diseases that can be changed by modifying one's environment, behavior, or lifestyle practices.

Examples: Modifiable risk factors for heart disease include cigarette smoking, sedentary lifestyle, and a diet high in fat, sugar, and salt, all of which can be modified to reduce the chances of early death from heart disease.

Morbidity

A departure from a state of health and well-being, measured by the extent of illness or disability among people in a given population over a specific period of time. Morbidity represents the number of people living with a disease, expressed as a rate or proportion of persons with the disease to the total population.

Mores

Strongly held norms or specific cultural expectations with a moral connotation, based on the values of the particular culture.

Mortality

The number of deaths that have occurred in a given time (e.g., within one year) or place (e.g., a specified population), usually expressed as a rate or proportion.

Mortality statistics are important to public health and health promotion in planning prevention programs for communities through providing information on causes of death and giving an indication of people's risk of dying from a particular disease during a defined period of time. Mortality data provide evidence of the frequency of a disease as it occurs in time, place, and persons and may be important in predicting disease trends.

Multiple Causation

A number of different causes. For example, a given disease may be the result of a combination of host-related factors linked to characteristics of the human population, agent-related factors associated with a specific cause, and environmental factors.

The idea underlying multiple causation is that disease, both infectious and chronic, is very complex and cannot be related to a single cause. To understand the process of a disease, one must look at a multiplicity of factors, such as accidents, violence, substance use and abuse, environmental decay, lack of health-promoting resources, and resources including time and place.

Example: Heart disease cannot be related to any one cause. There are multiple risk factors to be considered, including hypertension; family history of heart disease; sedentary lifestyle; social pressures; cigarette smoking; and dietary excesses of salt, saturated fats, and cholesterol-laden foods.

Multiple Determinants of Health

The concept that health, a basic human right, does not just happen but is determined by multiple factors. These factors may include social, psychological, personal, physical, and spiritual resources and capabilities; factors such as adequate food, shelter, education, health, and social services and access to these services; health behaviors and coping skills; income and employment; race, social support, social capital, and genetics; a supportive health environment; and public policy that enhances people's ability to control their own health by taking appropriate action.

N

Needs Assessment

A formal process of identifying problems and needs in a target population so as to make decisions, determine priorities, set objectives, and explore alternative approaches or methods to aid in the planning and implementation of programs. Needs assessment is the study of the setting in which, for example, a health education program is to be conducted and is used largely in the first steps of planning to help determine how capable the community is in addressing its health needs.

Needs assessment involves making a social diagnosis to determine the social concerns of the people for whom the program is to be developed, an epidemiological diagnosis to review health statistics in an effort to decide on the most appropriate program to develop, a behavioral diagnosis to identify behavioral factors or barriers to health, an educational diagnosis to ascertain participants' knowledge of the issue and their health-related skills, and an administrative diagnosis to assess available resources necessary to achieve the program objectives (Butler, 1994; Green & Kreuter, 1999; Windsor, Baranowski, Clark, & Cutter, 1994).

The needs assessment process involves gathering data concerning the perceived health needs of the population to determine current and existing conditions; analyzing the data by looking at the incidence and prevalence of problems, including mortality and morbidity statistics; and establishing priorities based on the ability to meet needs and available resources. See *PRECEDE/PROCEED Model*.

Noise Pollution

Excessive amounts of noise or sound that may lead to hearing loss and may also affect a person's health both physically and psychologically.

Nominal Group Process

A technique for generating and prioritizing needs or problems by asking group members to list problems in round-robin fashion, followed by rank ordering to determine the most pressing concerns.

Notifiable Disease

Any infectious disease that must be reported by health officials to public health departments for public health reasons including protection of the public's health.

O

Objective

A precise statement of what we intend to accomplish, stating exactly where we are going and indicating how we will know when we have arrived. In health education, objectives are quantified statements of desired health status, specific activities to be completed, or health system performance to be achieved within a specified time period. Objectives are usually measurable and embody the aims or goals of an activity. Objectives include outcomes to be achieved, how they will be observed, and criteria for deciding whether or not they were achieved. Achievement is reflected in standards of performance and evaluation. See *Behavioral Objective, Educational Objective,* and *Program Objective.*

Occupational Health

Concerns of health and health issues related to the work environment. Occupational health encompasses a person's ability to adjust to the work environment and to people who work in the same environment.

Occupational Injury

Any injury that occurs on the job or in the work environment.

Opinion Leader

A person in a community who is identified as playing a key role in the understanding of innovations such as new public health ideas, policy actions, and technology and communicating information to community groups. Opinion leaders are important for the success of many community health programs.

Oral Rehydration Therapy

Administration by mouth of a solution of sodium concentrates, sugar, and water to prevent dehydration in children with diarrheal problems and concomitant vomiting. The most common components of the solution are sodium, potassium, and glucose. Oral rehydration therapy is most often used in international settings where physicians or nurses are not always readily available and is the primary treatment for preventing death from dehydration. The solution can also be prepared at home (Graeff, Elder, & Mills-Booth, 1993; King, Glass, Bresee, & Duggan, 2003).

Outcome Evaluation

Assessment of the long-term effects of a program, for example, by observing health status and quality-of-life indicators in the earliest stages of a program and comparing them with the outcome. Outcome evaluation helps determine whether or not the program met the stated short- and long-term goals and objectives (Green & Kreuter, 1999; Windsor, Baranowski, Clark, & Cutter, 1994).

Outcome evaluation (sometimes referred to as *impact evaluation*) is important to health educators because it helps document the degree to which programs were conducted in accordance with the written plan, including goals, objectives, and results or benefits to participants. See *Impact Evaluation* and *Program Evaluation*.

Example: An outcome evaluation might ask, "Was there a reduction in maternal mortality rates in the priority population as a result of the program?"

P

Pandemic

An outbreak of a disease affecting people and sometimes animals that is felt over an extensive geographical area.

Paradigm

A broader concept than a theory that provides a way of looking at and interpreting subject matter, a view of the world, a particular field of study, a course of study, or a problem under investigation. In health education, a paradigm is a model or framework that provides a context from which research is conducted, knowledge is accumulated, and boundaries are created in effort to find answers or solve problems. See *Theory*.

Passive Intervention

An initiative, ordinarily sponsored by the government, for health promotion, education, and disease prevention interventions that do not necessarily require direct individual involvement.

Example: Fortification of certain foods with vitamin B_{12}

Passive Smoking

The inhalation of cigarette smoke or environmental tobacco by nonsmokers who are close to or in the same room with smokers or the burning ends of cigarettes.

Patient Education

Any planned learning experience using a combination of teaching methods, counseling, and behavior modification techniques to influence the knowledge and health behavior of patients. Patient education is concerned with helping patients learn how to care for themselves and to participate in decisions about their health care. It helps prepare patients to deal with changes in medical care.

The greater part of patient education is done by nurses, although health educators and preventive medicine professionals are often employed to plan and teach patients about exercise regimens, dietary changes, and inherited traits of disease to help them reduce stress and cope with their illnesses.

Perceived Barriers

Factors in the environment or community that a person believes may prevent him or her from carrying out a behavior, accessing health care, or attending a program. The individual may decide that the program is too expensive, the procedure is too unpleasant or dangerous, or there is too much inconvenience involved to take any action for improving his or her health.

Perceived Health

A person's day-to-day health as interpreted by the individual on the basis of knowledge and information gained from education, cultural, social, economic, family, and environmental situations.

Performance Indicators

A series of specific concepts and skills intended for fourth-, eighth-, and eleventh-grade students meant to help health educators and teachers focus on the most essential knowledge and skills basic to the development of health literacy among students. They also are intended to serve as a blueprint for organizing student assessment. In higher education, performance indicators include assessment of both institution and student, looking at student retention and completion rates; teaching quality; learning outcomes; and performance of graduates. See *Health Education Standards*.

Physical Education

Teaching that focuses on corporeal activity, fitness, and wellness in individuals, groups, communities, schools, and colleges. It includes the development of movement skills, knowledge, self-image, and social development and interaction, as well as strategies to promote confidence, self-assessment, cooperation, and independent learning.

Pilot Testing

Trying out research interventions and methods or health education programs and projects to uncover problems before the actual program or research project is launched.

A pilot test may involve a data collection instrument administered to a small test group as similar as possible to the group on which the instrument will actually be used. The pilot test enables the researcher to assess the clarity, sequence, length, and appropriateness of the instrument.

Pilot tests are designed to study data, collect information, and test an instrument (questionnaire) during the development phase of a research or intervention, to improve and document feasibility of program implementation; behavioral impact; and appropriateness of content, methods, materials, or instruments.

Example: Prior to conducting research, when a questionnaire is developed, a few copies (up to fifty, depending on the proposed sample size) are sent to a sample of people with the same characteristics as the intended research population. Responses enable a review of the questionnaire for appropriateness.

Planned Approach to Community Health (PATCH)

A program developed by the Centers for Disease Control and Prevention (CDC) in 1983 as a model to guide community organizers in the development and implementation of health promotion. The program was designed to help communities analyze their needs and plan, implement, and evaluate health promotion programs. Currently, the CDC provides technical assistance and training to states rather than communities. The approach is to begin at the grassroots level, such as a small group of people in a community who are interested in improving the overall health of community members. Using a team approach, people in the community make the decisions and do the work, with technical assistance from state or local health departments and the CDC. PATCH has its foundation in the diagnostic planning principles of the PRECEDE/PROCEED Model and is aimed at translating complex methods of health education practice and intervention to communities and community organizations through health agencies. Training for PATCH is at the community level. See *Community Organization* and *PRECEDE/PROCEED Model;* see also *Centers for Disease Control and Prevention* in Part Two.

Policy

A set of objectives or a course of action considered advantageous or expedient in guiding the activities of an organization and providing authority for allocation of resources (Harrington & Estes, 2001). Depending on the organization or level of employment, health educators may not be actively involved in policymaking but may significantly influence policymakers. Health educators should, whenever possible, participate in policy development regarding health issues.

Policy Intervention

The use of policy regulations to address problems and bring about change, ordinarily involving laws, policies, regulations, and formal and informal rules and understandings intended to guide individual and collective behavior (Wallack, Dorfman, Jernigan, & Themba, 1993).

Population at Risk

People in a community who might have been exposed to a disease or other health problem and become susceptible, whether or not they are affected by the disease or health condition.

Population Attributable Risk

The number of excess cases of people with a disease in a population that can be attributed to a particular risk factor. Population attributable risk is a joint function of relative risk, the prevalence of a risk factor in the population, and the absolute risk of disease.

Example: Roughly 135,000 people die each year from lung cancer in the United States. The relative risk of lung cancer in smokers is 10 to 1; one-third of the American population smokes, so 101,000 lung cancer deaths per year are attributable to smoking. Alternatively, there might have been 101,000 fewer deaths if no one smoked.

Population-Based Health Education

"Health education interventions designed to promote health and prevent disease within groups and communities rather than focusing on individuals" (2000 Joint Committee on Health Education Terminology, 2001, p. 9).

Population Health

"Health status of people who are not organized and have no identity as a group or locality and the actions and conditions to promote, protect, and preserve their health" (McKenzie, Pinger, & Kotecki, 2002, p. 606).

Postsecondary Health Education Program

"A planned set of health education policies, procedures, activities, and services that are directed to students, faculty, and/or staff of colleges, universities, and other higher education institutions" (1990 Joint Committee on Health Education Terminology, 1991, p. 107). Health education at this level may include some general health courses for students, health promotion activities targeting employees and students, health services, and appropriate preparation of health educators and other professionals. The intent is to promote, improve, and protect the health of students as well as that of faculty and staff.

Posttest

An evaluation instrument that provides the educator with data that are interpreted in terms of the learning that is assumed to have taken place over a given period of time. It measures learning progress or behavior change over a given period and is given after a pretest was administered.

PRECEDE/PROCEED Model

A model prescribing eight steps or phases in planning, implementing, and evaluating a health promotion program:

1. Social assessment (assessment of quality of life)
2. Epidemiological assessment (use of epidemiological data to determine health problems)
3. Behavioral and environmental assessment (identifying health-related and non-health-related behaviors or factors in the environment)
4. Educational and ecological assessment (sorting factors that may potentially affect health behaviors)
5. Administrative and policy assessment (resource assessment for program implementation)
6–8. Implementation and evaluation of program

The acronym PRECEDE stands for the diagnostic phases of health education and promotion planning: "*p*redisposing, *r*einforcing, and *e*nabling *c*onstructs in *e*ducational *d*iagnosis and *e*valuation." This framework also helps health planners identify priorities and set objectives for program implementation and evaluation and include factors involved in implementation, which is referred to as PROCEED: *p*olicy, *r*egulatory, and *o*rganizational *c*onstructs in *e*ducational and *e*nvironmental *d*evelopment (Green & Kreuter, 1999).

Predictable Variable

In considering the association between cause and effect, the variable that precedes the other (or is presumed on biologic grounds to be antecedent).

Example: In the relationship between gender and occurrence of heart disease, gender is the predictor variable.

Predisposing Factor

An independent construct such as knowledge, attitudes, beliefs, values, and perceptions in a person or population that motivates behavior before the behavior actually occurs. These characteristics are considered antecedents to the occurrence of particular health-related behaviors (Green & Kreuter, 1999).

Examples: If an AIDS prevention education program is being planned for teenagers, predisposing factors that may be considered are teenagers' knowledge about AIDS, attitudes toward behavior that put them at risk, beliefs about how the disease is transmitted, and their perception of themselves as being invincible.

Pretest

In formative research or program design, a process of systematically gathering target audience reactions to messages and materials before they are produced in final form or measuring a variable before an intervention begins. Various techniques are used to determine, for example, the relevance of a program to its audience, the relevance of a questionnaire to its intended target group, or the level of existing knowledge of topic prior to a presentation, lecture, workshop, or course of study. The pretest is administered before implementation of the program, experiment, or research.

Prevalence

A measure of the extent of a health problem or disease in a population based on the total number of existing cases at a given time. From a public health perspective, prevalence is of great importance, because health care services may be distributed according to the existing health and disease status of the population.

Prevention

In the health field, specific actions taken to identify risk factors, prevent or reduce the development of a health problem or condition, and minimize any damage that may have resulted from a previous condition. There are three levels of prevention: primary (reducing exposure to the disease before it occurs), secondary (early detection and prompt treatment to deter further decay), and tertiary (interventions to limit further disability and early death). See *Primary Prevention*, *Secondary Prevention*, and *Tertiary Prevention*.

Preventive Services

Interventions provided primarily in clinical settings. Among the current priority areas are maternal and infant health, cancer, heart disease and stroke, HIV infection, sexually transmitted diseases (STDs), and immunization for infectious diseases.

Preventive services may involve early prenatal care to prevent babies with low birth weight and infant deaths; reduction of tobacco use, dietary fat intake, and high blood pressure in an effort to prevent heart disease and stroke; mammography, clinical breast examination, Pap tests, fecal occult blood tests, and digital rectal examinations to detect and treat cancers before they spread; increasing use of condoms among sexually active men with multiple partners to prevent STDs; and increasing immunization to help eliminate infectious diseases such as tuberculosis, diphtheria, polio, rubella, and measles.

Primary Health Care

The first level of contact for individuals, family, and community to obtain basic health care that does not necessarily require a physician. It is essential health care provided to communities by means acceptable to them, with their participation, and at an affordable cost.

Primary health care includes health education, environmental sanitation (particularly food and water), promotion of nutrition, maternal and child health programs, immunization, family planning, and appropriate treatment of common diseases and injuries. Primary health care, mostly seen in developing countries and poorer nations, is usually an integral part of the country's health care system. In setting up a primary health care program, goals are developed, budgets identified and assigned, strategies are formulated, and pilot projects are undertaken.

Personnel for primary health care are auxiliary workers, health educators, dental hygienists, nurses, midwives, nurse practitioners, village health workers, and occasionally a physician or dentist. Primary health care may vary from country to country, depending on needs and resources.

Primary Prevention

The intervention or use of specific strategies and programs to reduce the occurrence of disease in a population. The first level of prevention, it is aimed at deterring disease before it occurs (Butler, 2000).

Much of primary prevention is accomplished through health promotion and education and certain environmental protection actions. Interventions may include water fluoridation to prevent dental decay, eradication of mosquitoes to prevent malaria, promoting sexual abstinence among teenagers to prevent HIV/AIDS transmission, and the wearing of safety equipment to prevent accidents when working with machinery.

Private Health Agency

A nongovernmental agency organized as a for-profit or nonprofit incorporated (voluntary), unincorporated (voluntary), or commercial organization concerned with health, health services, and health education at the primary, secondary, and tertiary levels of prevention. See *Voluntary Health Organization or Agency.*

Examples: American Heart Association, National Dairy Council.

Process Evaluation

The study of program implementation to detect problems early on and determine whether the program strayed from the protocol. Assessing the materials used, program personnel performance, how communication is disseminated, quality of professional practice, and services through observation or periodic surveys assists in making changes or adjustments for successful completion of the program.

Process evaluation is an ongoing examination of what is delivered and how it is delivered and includes program conception, program staff, methods, activities, and effectiveness and efficiency in reaching the target group or population.

Process evaluation is "designed to document the degree to which program procedures were conducted according to a written program plan: How much of the intervention was provided, to whom, when, and by whom?" (Windsor, Baranowski, Clark, & Cutter, 1994, p. 14). See *Evaluation* and *Program Evaluation*.

Professional Development

Educational and learning activities that take place after a health professional or health educator has attained a level of professional preparation for the purpose of maintaining, improving, or enhancing competency in the field of study.

Program Evaluation

Appraisal of a program to demonstrate its worth or effectiveness and to make recommendations for improvements. Program evaluation helps in making comparisons with different types of programs, looking at achievements, cost-effectiveness, appropriateness, and if funded, whether requirements for funding were met. Also known as *assessment*. See *Evaluation*.

Program Implementation

The execution or carrying out of a planned program, when decisions are put into actions.

Program Management

Procedures or strategies set in place for regular monitoring of program activities that ensure that the stated objectives (including process objectives) are met, resources are appropriately and judiciously utilized, and staff are routinely supervised.

Program Objective

A specific measurable statement of a desired program outcome. Program objectives should be realistic and consistent with the policies and procedures of the organization or community agency sponsoring the program.

Example: "By the end of the program, participants will be able to list evaluation methodologies appropriate to health education programs."

Program Planning

The process in which needs (real or perceived) are assessed, identified, analyzed, and defined; problems are diagnosed; resources are allocated; and barriers are assessed in order to achieve objectives. Then a program or plan of solution is designed to reflect the needs assessment. The PRECEDE/PROCEED Model can be used.

In the health education field, program planning begins with an interest in a specific health issue and is concerned with the group at risk, incidence and prevalence rates, specific behaviors to be targeted, and how these may change or be addressed with a health education intervention. Program planning is also concerned with resources (materials, personnel, money, time) that are available or can be made available to put the intervention into effect (Green & Kreuter, 1999; Windsor, Baranowski, Clark, & Cutter, 1994).

Program Sustainability

Continuation of a program or project beyond its completion; particularly after a funding cycle has ended. This involves taking action steps to gain community support and commitment, collaboration, providing tools and necessary information, and putting strategies in place to support and continue the program on a more permanent basis.

Psychomotor Domain

A category for classifying learning objectives related to neuromuscular coordination, including physical skills, habits, and general practices.

Example: Individuals develop appropriate health behavior patterns, such as scheduling an annual Pap test, having an annual physical or dental examination, or conducting routine breast self-examinations.

Psychosomatic Illness

Bodily symptoms resulting from mental conflict rather than from a physiological basis. A mind-body disease relationship clearly exists, but this is mainly due to personality. People may think they are sick and may even show symptoms when tests reveal that there is nothing physiologically wrong. It is estimated that nearly half of all people seeking medical attention suffer from some psychosomatic disorder associated with emotional stress (Bedworth & Bedworth, 1992). Health education and promotion endeavors should consider this factor in approaches to help people.

Public Health

Preventing disease, prolonging life, and promoting health and efficiency through organized community efforts for the sanitation of the environment, control of communicable infections, education in personal hygiene, organization of medical and nursing services, and development of the social machinery to ensure everyone a standard of living adequate for the maintenance of health.

Public health focuses primarily on the health of populations, communities, and organizations rather than individuals and is committed to social responsibility. Usually, public health is concerned with a health problem, based on the assumption that the social, physical, and political environments play major roles in the amelioration of the problem.

Public health, a major force in keeping the nation well, recognizes personal health habits as a strong influence in the causes of morbidity and mortality. The key components of public health include health policy, epidemiology, nutrition, occupational and environmental health, health education, control of communicable disease, health services administration, and injury control. Public health is also devoted to primary prevention (avoiding disease before it occurs).

Public Health Practice

The provision of health services aimed at protecting health, promoting health, and preventing disease that involve direct contact with the public or communities, including private and governmental, national, and international organizations, agencies, and other health care settings. The intent is to assist in solving current public health problems and to form linkages between public health educational institutions and public or community sites.

The U.S. Department of Health and Human Services has identified ten essential services used to facilitate public health practice at the federal, state, and local levels: monitoring community health status; diagnosing and investigating community health problems and hazards; educating and informing as well as empowering people about important health issues; identifying and resolving health problems by mobilizing community partners; developing policies and plans in an effort to support individual and community health efforts; protecting health and ensuring safety through the enforcement of laws and regulations; providing linkages between people and health services; ensuring that a competent and personal workforce exists; employing evaluation techniques to improve quality, accessibility, and effectiveness of health care services; and continuing research efforts for new and innovative solutions to health care problems.

Public Health Professional

"A person educated in public health or a related discipline who is employed to improve health through a population focus" (Gibbic, Rosenstock, & Hernandez, 2003, p. 4).

Public Service Announcement

Any message intended for the public disseminated without charge by the media (print, television, radio) to promote health programs and activities intended for community involvement or participation.

Q

Qualitative Approach

A research method that employs descriptive methodology to collect data such as interviews, case studies, focus groups, and observations. It is a more naturalistic approach than the traditional quantitative approach to research (Steckler, McLeroy, Goodman, Bird, & McCormick, 1992; Windsor, Baranowski, Clark, & Cutter, 1994).

The qualitative approach follows an inquiry process of understanding social or human problems, usually conducted in a natural setting and including the reporting of informants' views. Using the qualitative approach, investigators interact with their study subjects, sometimes living with them in the community and observing them over a period of time. Facts are then reported from evidence gathered. The style used to report the findings may be different from that of traditional research, less formal, more personal, and based on terms that emerge during the study. See *Quantitative Approach.*

Quality Assurance

A formal process of assessing the quality of a program or project and making improvements to assure providers, financiers such as funding agencies, and consumers that professional activities have been performed appropriately. Quality assurance, as defined by Windsor, Baranowski, Clark, and Cutter (1994), is "the appropriateness of a set of professional procedures for a problem and objectives to be achieved" (p. 101).

Quality assurance consists of observing and assessing program procedures, including how the staff carry out the program. A quality assurance investigator examines events that took place, such as problems that arose during program development and implementation, and demands proper documentation of the competency of key personnel or providers.

Quality of Life

People's perception as to whether or not their needs are being satisfied and opportunities are being presented that allow for the achievement of happiness and fulfillment. It is used as a public health measure ("Quality of Life," 1994).

The quality-of-life assessment helps health professionals see the situation through the eyes of community members and understand what is important to them. Health education is aimed at improving the quality of life through the promotion of healthy conditions, but to be effective, community members must view these conditions as important.

The quality of life may be assessed through simple questionnaires, face-to-face interviews, or focus groups or forums to obtain a consensus as to priorities. Discussions are important because even in the same community, people may have different perceptions on quality-of-life concerns owing to different cultural backgrounds, interests, and perceived needs. See *PRECEDE/PROCEED Model* and *Social Assessment*.

Quantitative Approach

A deductive method (applying a generally accepted principle to an individual case) that employs hard data, such as counts, ratings, scores, or classifications, to summarize findings.

The quantitative approach to research, as opposed to the qualitative method, is based on the testing of a theory composed of variables. Quantitative research involves measurements with numbers, statistical procedures, and data analysis in order to determine whether or not the predictions of a theory or hypothesis are true.

The quantitative method is a more traditional approach to research than qualitative approaches. The researcher remains distant from and independent of the subjects being studied, controls for bias, selects systematic samples, and tests hypotheses (chosen prior to the study) to determine cause and effect. The quantitative approach helps researchers develop certain generalizations (which contribute to theories) and enables them to predict and explain results (Creswell, 1994; Windsor, Baranowski, Clark, & Cutter, 1994). See *Qualitative Approach.*

Quasi-Governmental Health Organization

An organization such as the American Red Cross that operates like a voluntary agency even though some of its responsibilities are assigned by the government.

R

Reciprocal Determinism

The concept that the environment can shape a person and that the person can shape the environment. Reciprocal determinism is the continuous shared interaction among a person's behavior, personality, life situations, and external environment; they all influence one another. See *Social Cognitive Theory*.

Reducing Health Disparities

Efforts through advocacy, health policy, improved health care practices, and improved health care access, including health insurance, education, and research, to narrow the gap between the differences in health status that exist among certain population groups in the United States. See *Health Disparities*.

Reinforcing Factor

A reward, feedback, punishment, or incentive that a learner receives from others subsequent to the adoption of a behavior—in the context of the health education field, a health behavior. Reinforcing factors contribute to the individual's persistence in the behavior and serve to strengthen the motivation. Reinforcing factors can include attitudes and behavior of health personnel, peers, employees, parents, and relatives.

Relapse Prevention

Any maintenance strategy used to prevent an individual from reverting to behaviors after recent lifestyle modification or behavior change. A program for relapse prevention may use self-control principles to help individuals cope with problems in the process of changing behavior.

Example: A person attends a smoking cessation program and quits smoking but may slip back into the smoking habit if not provided with a maintenance program.

Relative Risk

The ratio of the incidence or chance of a disease or health problem in individuals exposed to a risk factor compared with the risk of disease or health in individuals without exposure. It is the relationship that exists between the risk of getting a disease when a risk factor is present and that of getting the same disease without the presence of the risk factor.

Examples: The relative risk of lung cancer for a forty-five-year-old heavy cigarette smoker compared with a nonsmoker may be about 10 to 1, and the relative risk of heart disease may be about 2 to 1.

Reliability

Consistency in the measurement of information or research results each time a study or experience is repeated. If an instrument (questionnaire or measurement tool) is reliable, it will give the same (or almost the same) results, but not perfect accuracy, every time it is used.

Resiliency

The combination of factors that contribute to survival and decisions related to health-promoting choices, especially in cases of individuals who display several risk factors that make healthy choices unlikely.

Retroactive Facilitation

The review of material or the discovery of new explicit relationships resulting in greater retention of a previous experience.

Retroactive Inhibition

The effect that present learning can have on the retention of previously learned material. New learning, or the accumulation of facts, about a basic food group, for example, may hinder the retention of previous learning about that food group, especially if there is some confusion about the previous information.

Risk Behaviors

Practices, habits, or actions that put individuals at risk for disease or health-related problems, including cigarette smoking, sexual intercourse at an early age, multiple sex partners, consumption of high-fat foods, driving without seat belts, riding a bicycle or motorcycle without a helmet, and domestic violence (Grunbaum & Basen-Engquist, 1993; "Quality of Life," 1994; Zimmerman & Olson, 1994).

Risk Communication

Dialogue or communication between health professionals and people in a community regarding health risks, including environmental health issues that may jeopardize health and ways to deal with them. Risk communication also covers risks related to genetics and choices that may follow.

Risk Factors

Social, environmental, and lifestyle or behavioral causes known to increase an individual's risk or probability of acquiring a specific disease or injury.

Risk Reduction

Decreasing factors that put individuals or communities at risk of developing a health problem or disease.

Role Delineation

The process of clarifying the role performed by health educators through the specification of responsibilities and functions and the identification of requisite skills and knowledge.

S

Sampling

Selecting a portion of a population for study that represents the target population as closely as possible and minimizes bias due to selection. The results of observations of this group then serves as the basis for arriving at general conclusions about the entire population.

Sampling is necessary to overcome the problem of representativeness in selecting a sample of a population. Selecting people (e.g., teenagers attending a clinic for sexually transmitted diseases) randomly or by a systematic method (e.g., every fifth teenager who visits the clinic) gives a basis for expecting the data to be representative of the population as a whole.

When an evaluation or survey research is being planned, one of the first concerns is the sample size and its selection. In selecting a sample, some random component should be included in order to generalize to the population being studied.

School-Based Health Services

Support services based at school to ensure access to health care for students. These services may include health clinics, child care, and appropriate social and health services. School-based health services may also include violence prevention; weight reduction, nutrition, and other health education services; acute care; laboratory services; health-screening examinations; and psychosocial services (Taras, 1994; Yates, 1994).

School Food Services

School-based services that provide meals to students that are nutritious, nutritionally balanced, affordable, and appealing. Included in school food services are nutrition education and the promotion of good eating habits among children and families.

School Health

A multiphasic program covering the physiological, sociological, psychological, and spiritual aspects of health in the school setting.

School health is concerned with health education (both formal and informal), instruction (a program of planned activities that takes place in the school), health services (rendered by a nurse or other health professional), and a healthful school environment (a safe and healthful climate and surroundings). School health is important because the health status of the students may affect their learning and their ability to achieve. Schools are expected to offer support, take responsibility for the children's health, and provide educational opportunities to help students live in and adjust to society. Schools have a unique opportunity to promote health and aid in the prevention of disease (Belzer & McIntyre, 1994; Cornacchia, Olsen, & Nickerson, 1991).

School Health Coordinator

"A certified or licensed professional at the state, district, or school level who is responsible for managing, coordinating, implementing, and evaluating all school health policies, activities, and resources" (2000 Joint Committee on Health Education Terminology, 2001, p. 9).

School Health Education

The component of the school health program (health services, healthful school environment, health instruction) that provides teaching and learning experiences. School health education is also concerned with developing, implementing, and evaluating planned instructional programs and activities that favorably influence knowledge, attitudes, habits, practices, appreciations, and conduct pertaining to the health of students. School health education is aimed at protecting and promoting health among students and school personnel. It is usually planned and conducted under the supervision of school personnel and with involvement of community health personnel (Hamburg, 1993; Schall, 1994).

See *Healthful School Environment, School Health Environment,* and *School Health Instruction.*

School Health Educator

A person with professional preparation in the field of school health education who meets the teaching requirements of his or her state and shows competency in developing, delivering, and evaluating curricula that will help enhance health knowledge, attitudes, and problem-solving skills for students and adults in the school setting.

School Health Environment

An important component of comprehensive school health education concerned with establishing a safe climate for children that enhances opportunities for learning. It includes site selection (away from landfills), school design, number of rest rooms, type of building, safe playgrounds, acceptable water supply, and other environmental concerns (Rudd & Walsh, 1993). See *Healthful School Environment* and *School Health.*

School Health Instruction

Teaching on the topics of personal health and hygiene, substance use and abuse, safety and accident prevention, family life, nutrition education, growth and development, disease prevention and control, and environmental health. Instructional methods must be appropriate to behavior change and outcome-oriented. See *School Health Education.*

School Health Services

Procedures to promote, appraise, and protect the health of schoolchildren. Services may be provided by physicians, nurses, teachers, dentists, dietitians, school counselors, and others (Brandon, 1993; Yates, 1994).

School health services provide first aid and care for students who may become injured or ill at school; immunization; and screening for dental caries, sickle cell anemia, and other conditions.

"School health services are that part of the school health program provided by physicians, nurses, dentists, health educators, other allied health personnel, social workers, teachers and others to appraise, protect and promote the health of students and school personnel. These services are designed to insure access to and the appropriate use of primary health care services, prevent and control communicable disease, provide emergency care for injury or sudden illness, promote and provide optimum sanitary conditions in a safe school facility and environment, and provide concurrent learning opportunities which are conducive to the maintenance and promotion of individual and community health" (1990 Joint Committee on Health Education Terminology, 1991, p. 106). See *School Health*.

Screening

Use of specific procedures to help determine if apparently well persons have a disease or are at high risk of having a disease. Screening is also performed to identify persons who may be considered high-risk individuals in order to carry out more definitive studies and to follow up a health condition.

Secondary Prevention

Any intervention strategy, such as case finding, screening, and treatment, intended to reduce the presence of an existing disease in a population, thus preventing further deterioration and early death.

Secondary prevention is concerned with early detection and prompt treatment of disease. The goal is to identify the disease at its earliest stage and apply appropriate treatments to limit its severity or diminish its impact. See *Prevention*.

Examples: Detecting breast cancer in its earliest stage (before metastasis, or spread) and intervening with treatment (surgery, chemotherapy); blood pressure screening and follow-up programs.

Secondhand Smoke

The smoke from cigarettes that is inhaled by nonsmokers; also known as *environmental tobacco smoke*.

Sedentary Behavior

Inactivity as a lifestyle behavior, characterized by opting to sit whenever there is an opportunity to do so instead of engaging in some form of activity.

Selective Prevention Intervention

An intervention "targeted to individuals or a subgroup of the population whose risk of developing substance abuse is significantly higher than average. The risk may be imminent or it may be a lifetime risk. The basis may be biological, psychological, or environmental" (U.S. Department of Health and Human Services, 2000, p. 265).

Self-Efficacy

A person's belief in his or her ability to perform a specific behavior. Self-efficacy is a construct that refers to the internal state that a person experiences, such as competence or capability to perform a desired task or behavior. See *Social Cognitive Theory*.

Example: (*format of a question used to determine self-efficacy*) "How confident are you that you could perform behavior X in situation Y?"

Self-Management

The concept that individuals can monitor a health behavior goal by keeping records of their own target behavior and factors associated with the behavior and provide self-rewards or reinforcements that will help increase the likelihood of achieving the goal. Self-management can be used in various health settings as part of a behavioral intervention strategy in health promotion programs.

Self-Regulation

The act or process of controlling health-threatening behavior by active recall of long-term consequences of the behavior. One of the aims of health promotion is to enable individuals to take control of or regulate their behavior. This involves identifying cues in the environment or in the individual's own thoughts and feelings that can help in controlling or regulating behavior.

Sensitivity

In the health field, a measurement used to evaluate diagnostic, prognostic, and screening tests to determine how well a test can discriminate between the diseased and the nondiseased. Sensitivity is indicated by the proportion of subjects with a disease who have a positive test result. It indicates how good a test is at identifying cases of the disease in a population or group. See *Specificity* and *Validity.*

Set Point Theory

The hypothesis that each person has an internally predetermined weight that the body attempts to maintain, despite efforts to change. The body's metabolism may even change to preserve the weight. Personal set points may differ from society's ideal weights. An understanding of this theory is important for health educators conducting programs designed to help individuals lose weight.

Sick-Role Behavior

Any activity undertaken for the purpose of getting well by persons who consider themselves to be ill or who were diagnosed with a medical problem. Sick-role behavior is similar to illness behavior. See *Illness Behavior.*

Example: Visiting a doctor for treatment and following the treatment protocol.

Social Assessment

"The assessment in both objective and subjective terms of high-priority problems or aspirations for the common good, defined for a population by economic and social indicators and by individuals in terms of their quality of life" (Green & Kreuter, 1999, p. 509).

Social Capital

"The processes and conditions among people and organizations that lead to accomplishing a goal of mutual social benefit, usually characterized by four interrelated constructs: trust, cooperation, civic engagement, and reciprocity" (Green & Kreuter, 1999, p. 509).

Social Cognitive Theory

A theory emphasizing the effect of the social environment and cognitive mediators such as beliefs on behavior and the reciprocal effect of behavior on environment and cognition. Social cognitive theory (formerly called *social learning theory*) explains learning as a reciprocal interaction among an individual's environment, thought processes, and behavior such that learning takes place through synthesized thoughts.

Social cognitive theory is applicable to health promotion in explaining and predicting behavior through key concepts such as incentives and outcome expectations. According to the theory, change is a function of expectations: for example, expectations of what may result from participating in a behavior change activity or one's ability to execute the behavior. Three key aspects to the theory are vicarious learning or imitation of the behavior, the use of symbols, and principles of self-management. See *Reciprocal Determinism* and *Self-Efficacy*.

Social Comparison Theory

A social-psychological theory suggesting that when people are confused about their internal state, they turn to others in order to interpret the situation.

Social Ecology

A way of looking at how people interact with their physical, social, and cultural environments. Ecology refers to the study of relationships between an organism (any individual life form) and its environment. The social ecology approach involves the identification of physical and social characteristics of the environment that may affect a person's health. These characteristics may include stress influenced by change of residence, noise in the neighborhood, social isolation, access to health care facilities, and safety. A consideration of these factors may lead to the development of health promotion programs focusing on change (Kaplan, Sallis, & Patterson, 1993).

Social ecology is useful to community health promotion in that it emphasizes the importance of environmental changes on health and can provide clues about the types of changes in the environment that facilitate both physical and emotional well-being of individuals and promote healthful behaviors (Stokols, 1992).

Social Inequality

Unequal social, educational, or economic opportunities given to people of a lower social status or position in a community, society, or group. In relation to health, it refers to unequal health treatment or programs available to people of different social positions in a society or community, as well as on an individual level.

Social Marketing

The consumer-driven application of marketing principles and techniques to program development, implementation, and evaluation in an effort to promote change or modification in health behavior (Kotler, Roberto, & Lee, 2002).

Applied to health promotion, social marketing requires program planners to provide products and services that are acceptable to the community. Products may include vegetarian cookbooks or pamphlets with the basic food guide information. Services may include the development of nutrition education programs and cooking classes.

The promotion aspect of the health program can be accomplished through the media, distribution of flyers, personal invitations, and word of mouth. The right place must also be found to make the products and services available to the community. Services and products can be offered at community centers, service clubs, tribal halls, churches, and worksites. In addition, health education materials can be made available at supermarkets, public libraries, clinics, and hospital waiting rooms.

Price includes the cost to produce and market the products and services (health education programs), taking into consideration time, transportation opportunities, and accessibility.

Social Networks

Chains of contacts established within a society to foster social relations and links between individuals for the purpose of providing social support for health and health issues and to reinforce behaviors that promote health and well-being. These networks give individuals access to other individuals, families, or groups who can help them cope with health problems or recovery from serious illness.

Social Support

Social contacts or interactions people maintain with others on a regular basis, along with family, friends, church members, and others they can rely on, care about, and love. Social support includes any kind of helping behavior that allow individuals to cope better when experiencing serious physical or psychological health problems and the satisfaction that is felt with social relationships.

It is believed that social relationships have an effect on health outcomes. A network of family, friends, and other social contacts may help ease stress and tensions resulting from sickness or injuries. People who experience good social support also seem to have healthier lifestyles. Positive social relationships may enhance health, including mental health outcomes, and have a protective effect for problems such as heart disease.

Building social support is a meaningful method of reinforcing self-directed health behaviors and can be informal, for example, asking a friend or family member to exercise with you or be your buddy during the course of a smoking cessation program (Fenlason & Beehr, 1994).

There are also more formal support groups for medical problems. Support groups initiated by the American Cancer Society for women who have undergone mastectomies or other treatments for breast cancer are one such example. These groups meet at scheduled times to offer support and learn more about the problem.

Socioeconomic Status (SES)

The social and economic positions of individuals or groups within a society. Those with very low socioeconomic status have the most difficulty accessing health care and usually experience the poorest health outcomes, while those of higher socioeconomic status experience ready access to health care and increased opportunities for engaging in health-promoting behaviors and therefore have better health outcomes.

Special Populations

People or groups within a community or population who might be more susceptible to certain health problems or be at greater risk for some diseases because of factors such as age, gender, previous health problems, occupation, conditions such as being pregnant, or lifestyle behaviors such as cigarette smoking that increase their risk for illness.

Specificity

A determination of how well a diagnostic, examination, or screening test discriminates between the diseased and the nondiseased. Specificity is expressed as the proportion of subjects without the disease who have a negative test result. It indicates how good a test is at identifying people without the disease in question.

Specificity and sensitivity are usually considered together as measures of validity. See *Sensitivity* and *Validity*.

Stages of Change

According to Prochaska and Di Clemente's transtheoretical model (Kaplan, Sallis, & Patterson, 1993), the sequence of stages a person goes through when attempting to change a behavior: precontemplation, contemplation, decision, action, and maintenance. People seem to move through an orderly sequence of change, some more rapidly than others. At each stage, different processes of change, or intervention approaches, are needed (Di Clemente et al., 1991; Kaplan et al., 1993).

In the precontemplation stage, people (precontemplators) have no intention to change a behavior but will at least become aware of the problem or behavior. In the contemplation stage, people (now contemplators) are thinking about making a change and are reevaluating their behavior. Then a decision is made. In the action stage, a person changes the behavior, and in the maintenance stage, the behavior change is sustained. See *Transtheoretical Model*.

Strategy

A plan of action consisting of broad approaches for achieving specific objectives, anticipating both barriers and resources.

Stress Response

Relatively stereotypical sets of interacting psychological and biological patterns that organisms exhibit in response to exposure to a stressor. When the body experiences certain stressful events, a stress response is induced if the person feels that he or she cannot cope with the adversity or stressor (Kaplan, Sallis, & Patterson, 1993). See *Stressor*.

Example: A stress response is created when a person adjusts to a stressor, such as the death of a loved one or recent news of test results indicating a disease such as cancer.

Stress-Buffering Model

The theory that social support absorbs the impact of stress. This model predicts that the relationship between social support and health outcome should occur only for individuals under high levels of stress and describes the protective effects that social support has on an individual.

According to this model, "social support may intervene in the pathway between the stressful event and the receiver" individual (McMahon, Schram, & Davidson, 1993, p. 242). In other words, friends may intervene by encouraging the person who is experiencing the stress, and the more positive the response, the more effective should be the outcome (McMahon et al., 1993; Ulbrich & Bradsher, 1993).

The model also indicates that when there is high stress and low social support, the result can be illness; but when there is high stress and high social support, the impact of stress is buffered or absorbed (DesCamp & Thomas, 1993; Revenson & Majerovitz, 1991). See *Social Support*.

Stressor

Any stimulus that makes demands on an individual requiring adaptation (e.g., making beneficial alterations to one's living conditions) or adjustment (modifying or altering one's behavior).

A stressor may be an event, physical or environmental, that triggers a response or threatens a person's existence and well-being and makes demands that require adaptation (Vlisides, Eddy, & Mozie, 1994; Whitehead, 1994).

Examples: Very cold weather, lack of sleep, sustained physical exercise, excessive noise, sorrow (from death of a family member), joy (news that you just won big money), fear, frustration

Summative Evaluation

An assessment conducted at the completion of a program to determine its effectiveness in achieving program objectives and whether the program should be continued. A summative evaluation also helps in measuring achievements, such as how many individuals actually changed a targeted behavior. See *Impact Evaluation, Outcome Evaluation,* and *Program Evaluation.*

Surveillance

In the health field, the process of monitoring diseases as they occur. It is the "continuing scrutiny of all aspects of occurrence and spread of disease that are pertinent to effective control" (Benenson, 1990, p. 507).

Example: The Centers for Disease Control and Prevention (CDC) is involved with surveillance of diseases and provide mortality and morbidity reports, reports of field investigations of epidemics, identification of infectious agents and new diseases, reports on effects of vaccines, information regarding immunity levels in population segments, and other relevant data. CDC surveillance summaries of diseases are published in the *Morbidity and Mortality Weekly Report.*

Survey

A method of collecting data from a group or population to estimate the norms and distribution of characteristics from a sample. Surveys usually employ instruments such as questionnaires, interviews, or direct observation.

The purpose of a survey is to obtain specific information from a specified group of people or population. A survey can be conducted in a variety of formats, such as face-to-face interviews, mailed or telephone questionnaires, focus groups, or direct observation.

Survey results can be used as baseline data for measuring change, for delineating and describing problems in a population, and for adding to the body of knowledge on the subject or issue under consideration.

System Barriers

"Conditions within a health care system that prevent people from accessing needed services or prevent health care providers from delivering those services. System barriers include physical, cultural, linguistic, and financial barriers as well as the availability of health care facilities or providers with special skills, such as eye, ear, nose, and throat specialists" (U.S. Department of Health and Human Services, 2000, p. 142).

Systems Approach

A school of thought postulating that most outcomes are the result of systems and not individuals. The systems approach attempts to improve the efficiency as well as the quality of a system by emphasizing how information flows and the interrelatedness of parts to the whole.

T

Target Population

A set of people or a community being targeted or focused on; also known as a *target group*. For example, if a prevention program is aimed at reducing the incidence of disease or addressing some health condition among a certain population, all efforts and communication will be designed to reach that particular group.

Example: Children between the ages of one and five years in Dallas, Texas, who are malnourished

Telehealth

The use of telephone, video, radio, and other electronic information systems to support and facilitate distance clinical health care, public health, patient education, health education, and health administration.

Tertiary Prevention

The third level or therapeutic stage of prevention. The first two levels are primary and secondary. Tertiary prevention employs intervention strategies directed at assisting diseased and disabled people in a population to reduce the impact of their disabilities.

Tertiary prevention relies more heavily on medical care and rehabilitation than on health promotion and education. Tertiary prevention may include patient education or cholesterol reduction for patients with heart disease. See *Primary Prevention* and *Secondary Prevention*.

Theory

A set of principles and concepts used to predict and explain a phenomenon, such as human behavior; an integrated set of propositions intended to give deeper understanding of a philosophy and provide a basis for explaining certain happenings of life.

In the health education field, theories are developed to explain the processes underlying learning and offer program planners a framework or guide in selecting interventions needed to accomplish stated goals and objectives. Large portions of health education and promotion programs are planned and evaluated on the basis of substantiated theories (Powers & Knapp, 1990). See *Theory of Planned Behavior* and *Theory of Reasoned Action*.

Theory of Planned Behavior

An extension of the theory of reasoned action that incorporates a person's attitudes toward a behavior. The use of this theory may have a significant impact on the development of health programs because it has been very successful in dealing with behaviors in which there is a conscious choice (Ajzen, 1991; Doll & Ajzen, 1992; Rodgers & Brawley, 1993; Wankel & Mummery, 1993). See *Theory of Reasoned Action*.

Theory of Reasoned Action

A social-psychological model of voluntary behavior based on the assumption that intentions are the most immediate influence on behavior. The theory emphasizes the role of personal intention in determining whether or not a behavior will occur.

According to this theory, intentions are influenced by attitudes and subjective norms, or perceptions of social pressures. Attitudes are determined by beliefs about the consequences of behavior, and subjective norms are affected by the actions of significant others.

The theory was developed to explain behavior and provide a framework for studying attitudes toward behavior. It was extended to include the concept of perceived control as a third influence on intentions. See *Behavioral Intention* and *Theory of Planned Behavior*.

Timeline

A working schedule developed and used in the planning and execution of a program or project to show the activities and the times when they are expected to be accomplished or developed during the course of the program. A timeline usually sets out the schedule of activities chronologically (by day, month, or year, depending on the period covered) from left to right. See *Gantt Chart*.

Triage

Prioritizing; grouping people or patients into categories of health needs or services to determine how resources will be allocated to them; evaluating patient conditions to establish their urgency and seriousness in order to prioritize the provision of health care or emergency attention.

Transtheoretical Model

A model developed by two psychologists, James Prochaska and Carlo Di Clemente, in 1984 to describe and explain stages that people go through during psychotherapy (Kaplan, Sallis, & Patterson, 1993). The model implies that as people pass through these stages of change (precontemplation, contemplation, decision, action, and maintenance), they may need different intervention approaches. Although not fully tested, the model has been useful in studying a variety of health behaviors, such as smoking. It has been applied in smoking cessation interventions and in alcohol treatment plans (Di Clemente & Hughes, 1990; Di Clemente et al., 1991). See *Stages of Change*.

U

Underinsured

Having some insurance coverage but not enough to cover all necessary health care services. As a result, underinsured patients are required to use their own money to cover expenses and may not be able to pay for the services they require.

Underserved

Having less access to health services or health information than the national average. The underserved may include persons of low socioeconomic status, persons with physical disabilities, or members of certain disadvantaged racial or ethnic groups.

Unintentional Injury

Any injury or impairment that is the result of an accident. Examples include injuries caused by motor vehicle collisions, fires, falls, drowning, and firearms.

Universal Preventive Interventions

Public health interventions that target entire populations instead of specific identified groups. These interventions may cost less and have a wider range of overall effectiveness because all who receive the intervention may benefit to some degree.

Unmodifiable Risk Factors

Factors that contribute to the development of diseases but cannot be modified or altered by behavior change or changes in the environment, such as age, gender, ethnicity, or race.

Example: A person born into a family where one parent or both parents had high serum cholesterol levels is at risk for the same high levels regardless of diet and exercise habits.

V

Validity

The degree to which a test or assessment measures what it is intended to measure. Using an acceptable (valid) instrument increases the chance of measuring what was intended (Vogt, 1993; Windsor, Baranowski, Clark, & Cutter, 1994).

Validity also describes the accuracy of a study or data collection instrument, in terms of both external and internal validity. It reflects the appropriateness or usefulness of specific inferences made from test scores or the quality of data derived from the use of an instrument (questionnaire).

Forms of validity regularly used in health education evaluation are content validity, criterion-related validity, and construct validity. See *Construct Validity, Content Validity, Criterion Validity, External Validity,* and *Internal Validity.*

Values

Highly esteemed cultural attitudes or beliefs shared by and transmitted among people who hold a common history or identity.

Values Clarification

Techniques that help learners clarify, define, and defend their true beliefs about moral, ethical, social, and other relationships. It emphasizes the processes that learners use to arrive at a value judgment and helps in the identification and clarification of their thinking regarding important issues without indoctrinating them or forcing them to take a position.

Vital Statistics

Records of births, deaths, marriages, and divorces reported to the United States government. These are excellent tools for monitoring a population's health over time. Vital statistics are also used in determining the allocation of health care funds in areas of great need. Furthermore, "a birth certificate establishes a person's legal existence and his or her basic legal relationships, including citizenship and parentage" (Scutchfield & Keck, 2003, p. 69).

Voluntary Health Organization or Agency

A nonprofit, nongovernmental association dedicated to providing health education or health services related to specific health concerns. Voluntary organizations are supported financially by contributions from individuals and agencies and depend on volunteers to perform much of the work.

Examples: American Heart Association, United Way, American Cancer Society

Vulnerable Populations

People who have several health as well as social needs and are at risk for being underrepresented or at higher risk because they do not have the same access to quality health care as the rest of the population. These may include some elderly people, substance abusers, people with mental health problems, migrant farmworkers, people infected with HIV, the poor, and the homeless.

W

Weight Cycling

The yo-yo diet syndrome of repeated weight losses and gains, which makes it more and more difficult to lose body fat or weight.

Wellness

A dimension of health that goes beyond the absence of disease or infirmity and includes the integration of social, mental, emotional, spiritual, and physical aspects of health. The concept of wellness was first introduced in the United States in the 1970s as an expanding experience of purposeful and enjoyable living. Wellness refers to a positive state, illness to a negative state (Butler, 2000; Green & Kreuter, 1999).

Wellness Centers

Facilities organized and operated mainly by health professionals, such as health education specialists, preventive care specialists, nurses, therapists, nutritionists, medical doctors with an interest in prevention, and health administrators, to provide people with learning opportunities about health behavior, risk reduction, and issues related to the health of the population. Learning opportunities may involve health education workshops, weight maintenance and control clinics, exercise demonstrations, cooking demonstrations, nutrition classes, and stress management programs.

Work Plan

A detailed description of the activities needed to reach stated objectives. Work plans must be written in a specific and detailed manner. They are tools that guide project implementation and should reflect the best projection of tasks, timelines, and evaluation strategies.

Worksite Health Promotion

Programs or interventions conducted at the place of employment or sponsored by employers to benefit employees and their families, a high percentage of whom may not otherwise participate in health promotion programs.

Health promotion at the worksite covers a wide variety of activities, including exercise and fitness, stress management, smoking cessation, and cholesterol reduction. Specific programs targeting women may include prenatal care, parenting, breast examinations, and mammograms.

Some worksite health promotion efforts may require that employees engage in behaviors that protect their health, such as wearing hard hats and not smoking or using alcohol on the job. The worksite offers enormous potential for health promotion, and employees as well as employers share in the benefits (Chenoweth, 1991; Modeste, 1994).

PART TWO

Health and Professional Organizations

N ote that most of the organizations and agencies listed here have coun-
terparts in other countries. There are also many additional health
agencies, both national and international, too numerous to mention here.

Action on Smoking and Health (ASH)

Action on Smoking and Health is a national charitable antismoking and
nonsmokers' rights organization. This organization serves members and
local groups. It focuses on publicizing the dangers of smoking through campaigns for a smoke-free public; promotes national No-Smoking Day; provides legal information to help nonsmokers protect their rights and health;
and liaises with health promotion organizations and private groups. ASH
also disseminates information related to smoking and health and monitors
scientific and trade publications. ASH publishes a biweekly information
bulletin and a quarterly supporter newsletter.

Address: 2013 H Street, N.W., Washington, DC 20006

Web Site: http://ash.org

Agency for Healthcare Research and Quality (AHRQ)

This agency, formerly the Agency for Health Care Policy and Research, was
created by Congress in 1989 within the Public Health Service. The agency
is federally funded, focuses on health services research including dissemination of findings, and is devoted specifically to prevention.

The purpose of the agency is to improve quality of health care, reduce
health care costs, and enhance the quality of life and safety of patient care
services through improved knowledge that can be used in meeting the health
care needs of society. AHRQ seeks to achieve its mission through several
broad goals: the promotion of improvements in clinical practice and patient

outcomes through more appropriate and effective health care services; the promotion of improvements in the financing, organization, and delivery of health care services; and the increase of access to high-quality care. The agency also sponsors individual and institutional National Research Service Awards, providing pre- and postdoctoral support for academics and for research concerning health services research methods and problems.

Address: 540 Gaither Road, Rockville, MD 20850

Agency for Toxic Substances and Disease Registry (ATSDR)

ATSDR works to prevent adverse human health effects and diminished quality of life that can result from exposure to hazardous substances in the environment. It is administered by the director of the Centers for Disease Control and Prevention (CDC) but is a separate agency.

ATSDR evaluates data and information on the release of hazardous substances into the environment. It assesses any current or future effects on public health, develops health advisories, and identifies studies or actions needed to evaluate and mitigate or prevent adverse human health effects. ATSDR increases an understanding of the relationship between exposure to hazardous substances and adverse effects on human health through epidemiology, surveillance, and other studies on toxic substances and their effects.

ATSDR monitors people's exposure to hazardous substances through a registry of people exposed to hazardous substances, serious diseases, and illnesses. In addition, it provides health-related support to states, local agencies, and health care providers in public health care emergencies that involve exposure to hazardous substances, health consultations, and training.

The agency develops and makes available to physicians and other health care providers materials on the health effects of toxic substances and maintains a list of sites that are closed or restricted to the public because of contamination. Summaries of such materials may also be made available to the public.

ATSDR identifies gaps in knowledge, initiates research in toxicology and health effects where needed, and conducts or sponsors applied research on the human health effects of hazardous substances released into the environment from waste sites or other hazardous wastes.

Address: 1600 Clifton Road, N.E., MS E-60, Atlanta, GA 30333

American Academy of Health Behavior

A society of researchers and scholars whose mission is to advance health education and health promotion through science-based research focusing on health behavior. The academy also seeks to disseminate research findings, collaborate with other professionals in research, and influence policies for acquiring resources for health behavior research.

Address: P.O. Box 31264, Charlotte, NC 28231

Web Site: http://www.aahb.org

American Alliance for Health, Physical Education, Recreation and Dance (AAHPERD)

AAHPERD is the largest organization of professionals whose role is to support and assist those in health, physical education, dance, and other specialties devoted to achieving a healthy lifestyle. The organization is made up of seven national associations:

1. American Association for Health Education (AAHE)—dedicated to improving human health through health education
2. American Association for Leisure and Recreation (AALR)—dedicated to enhancing the quality of life of the American people through the promotion of creative and meaningful leisure and recreation experiences; focuses on practitioners and educators as well as students
3. American Association for Active Lifestyles and Fitness (AAALF)—dedicated to serving professionals who conduct physical activity and fitness programs; advocates for populations that are underserved
4. National Association for Girls and Women in Sports (NAGWS)—fosters quality and equality in sports, including funding for girls

and women, and serves those who coach, teach, and administer sports

5. National Association for Sport and Physical Education (NASPE)—devoted to improving the total sports and physical education experience in the United States through the enhancement of knowledge and professional practice and the scientific study and dissemination of research-based findings

6. National Dance Association (NDA)—dedicated to promoting the development and implementation of knowledge and sound professional practices in dance education

7. Research Consortium (RC)—dedicated to furthering and promoting research and publications and the exchange of ideas among professionals in health education, recreation, athletics, exercise, and dance

Address (AAHPERD and Affiliates): 1900 Association Drive, Reston, VA 22091

American Association for H ealth Education (AAHE)

The American Association for Health Education (AAHE), formerly known as the Association for the Advancement of Health Education, is the oldest and largest health education association. It is one of seven associations that make up the American Alliance for Health, Physical Education, Recreation and Dance (AAHPERD) and focuses on health educators and other professionals concerned with the prevention, protection, preservation, and improvement of health through education and other strategies. AAHE is a national professional membership organization representing thousands of health educators and health promotion specialists who work in schools, colleges and universities, medical care facilities, community and public health agencies, and business and industry.

AAHE members benefit from a subscription to the *Journal of Health Education,* the *American Journal of Health Promotion,* and *HE-XTRA,* a newsletter from the national AAHE office reporting on news and current events in health education. Members also benefit from conferences, conventions, and leadership opportunities.

Address: 1900 Association Drive, Reston, VA 22091

Web Site: http://www.aahe.org

American College Health Association (ACHA)

ACHA is a professional organization made up of individuals and institutions of higher education addressing health problems such as teenage pregnancy, sex education, AIDS issues, school health education and services, and other health-related issues in the academic community. The association promotes continuing education, research, and program development primarily for schools and educational institutions.

Address: P.O. Box 28937, Baltimore, MD 21090

Web Site: http://www.acha.org

American College of Preventive Medicine (ACPM)

ACPM was established in 1954 as a national professional society for physicians committed to disease prevention and health promotion. Its members are engaged in preventive medicine practice, teaching, and research. Specialists in preventive medicine are uniquely trained in both clinical medicine and public health. Physicians trained in preventive medicine can be found working in primary care settings and managed care organizations, in public health and government agencies, in workplaces, and in academia, attempting to reduce the risks of disease, both in individuals and in groups within the population.

Address: 1307 New York Avenue, N.W., Suite 200, Washington, DC 20005

Web Site: http://www.acpm.org

American College of Sports Medicine (ACSM)

ACSM's mission is to promote and integrate scientific research, education, and practical applications of sports medicine and exercise science to maintain and enhance physical performance, fitness, health, and quality of life.

ACSM was founded in 1954. Since that time, members have applied their knowledge, training, and dedication in sports medicine and exercise science to promote healthier lifestyles for people around the globe.

ACSM continues to grow and prosper both nationally and internationally and is the largest sports medicine and exercise science organization in the world. Its members are committed to diagnosing, treating, and preventing sports-related injuries and the advancement of the science of exercise.

Address: 401 West Michigan Street, Indianapolis, IN 46202 *or* P.O. Box 1440, Indianapolis, IN 46206

Web Site: http://www.acsm.org

American Federation of Aging Research (AFAR)

AFAR supports biomedical research aimed at promoting healthier aging and provides opportunities for the interchange of knowledge and ideas about aging and health among physicians and scientists. It provides a forum for researchers to discuss the findings of aging research and ways of disseminating findings to the scientific and general public.

Address: 70 West Fortieth Street, 11th Floor, New York, NY 10018

Web Site: http://www.afar.org

American Public Health Association (APHA)

APHA, founded in 1872, is the largest public health organization in the world and is committed to the protection and promotion of personal and environmental health and the prevention of disease.

APHA represents all disciplines and specialties of public health and is active in policy development, setting public health practice standards, and special projects. The association plans annual conferences for the continuing professional development of its members as it brings together professionals from academia, research, administration, health service providers, and other health workers. The Public Health Promotion and Education and

School Health Education and Services sections are especially relevant to the concerns of health educators.

APHA is responsible for the publication of the *American Journal of Public Health* and a newsletter, *The Nation's Health.*

Address: 800 I Street, N.W., Washington, DC 20001

Web Site: http://www.apha.org

American School Health Association (ASHA)

ASHA is the primary professional organization concerned with issues related to school-age children. School health services, healthful school environment, and comprehensive school health education are key areas of concern.

ASHA publishes the *American Journal of School Health.*

Address: P.O. Box 708, Kent, OH 44240

Web Site: http://www.ashawed.org

Association of Reproductive Health Professionals (ARHP)

ARHP was founded in 1963 as an arm of the Planned Parenthood Federation of America but became an independent entity in 1972. It is a nonprofit membership association composed of highly qualified and committed experts in the field of reproductive health, including physicians, advanced practice clinicians such as nurse practitioners, nurse midwives, physician assistants, researchers, educators, pharmacists, and other professionals in reproductive health. ARHP and its members provide reproductive health services or education, conduct reproductive health research, or influence reproductive health policy. The organization reaches a broad range of health care professionals in the United States and abroad with education and information about reproductive health science and practice.

Address: 2401 Pennsylvania Avenue, N.W., Suite 350, Washington, DC 20037

Web Site: http://www.arhp.org

Association of Teachers of Preventive Medicine (ATPM)

ATPM is the national association supporting educators and researchers in health promotion and disease prevention. Since 1942, ATPM members have been in the forefront of advancing, promoting, and supporting health promotion and disease prevention in the education of physicians and other health professionals. ATPM members include physicians, nurses, public health professionals, and health services researchers, as well as institutional members such as academic departments and programs, health agencies, and schools of public health.

Address: 1660 L Street, N.W., Suite 208, Washington, DC 20036

Web Site: http://www.atpm.org

Bureau of Alcohol, Tobacco and Firearms (BATF)

BATF is a federal law enforcement entity within the U.S. Department of the Treasury responsible for regulating tobacco and alcohol and for reducing violent criminal activity and violence through law enforcement and community outreach. The bureau strives to foster public safety through a trained workforce.

Web Site: http://www.aft.gov

Canadian Council for Tobacco Control (CCTC)

The Canadian Council for Tobacco Control (formerly the Canadian Council on Smoking and Health) was founded in 1974 by nongovernmental organizations focusing on tobacco use in Canada. The council is dedicated to diminishing the adverse impact of tobacco products on Canadians and is committed to disseminate information on tobacco, to raise public awareness regarding the dangers of smoking, and to lobby for smoke-free public areas.

Address: 75 Albert Street, Suite 508, Ottawa, Ontario, Canada K1P 5E7

Web Site: http://www.cctc.ca

Canadian Public Health Association (CPHA)

CPHA is a not-for-profit voluntary association for health professionals. It supports health and social programs nationally and internationally. The association represents public health in Canada with links to the international public health community and provides members with an opportunity to speak out on broader public health issues. It aims at improving and maintaining personal and community health according to the public health principles of disease prevention, health promotion and protection, and healthy public policy.

CPHA is responsible for several publications, including the *Canadian Journal of Public Health,* a monthly professional journal, and a quarterly magazine titled *CPHA Health Digest.*

Web Site: http://www.cpha.org

Center for the Advancement of Health

The Center for the Advancement of Health provides leadership to ensure that money is invested in health research. The center is involved with translating health research findings into policy, as well as practice, and fostering alliances between research scientists and policymakers. It strives to communicate the best and most recent research findings and needs through its publication, *Health Behavior News Service.*

Address: 2000 Florida Avenue, N.W., Suite 210, Washington, DC 20009

Web Site: http://www.cfah.org.

Centers for Disease Control and Prevention (CDC)

CDC was established as the Communicable Disease Center in 1946 in Atlanta, Georgia, and has directed efforts toward preventing diseases such as malaria, polio, smallpox, toxic shock syndrome, Legionnaires' disease, AIDS, bioterrorism, and other health issues.

CDC is the leading federal agency for protecting the health and safety of people nationally and globally and is concerned with health education and promotion activities such as chronic disease prevention and control, tobacco use prevention and control, and injury prevention and control. CDC is also involved in health surveillance and selected treatment activities that support prevention.

According to CDC advertising, the mission of the agency is to promote health and quality of life by preventing and controlling disease, injury, and disability. Its mission is accomplished through national and international leadership; applied epidemiology, laboratory, and behavioral research; building the public health system through technical and financial assistance and training; setting standards and guidelines; and surveillance and data analysis. Research findings and surveillance data are published in the *Morbidity and Mortality Weekly Report*.

Address: 1600 Clifton Road N.E., Atlanta, GA 30333

Web Site: http://www.cdc.gov

Coalition of National Health Education Organizations (CNHEO)

CNHEO is a nonpartisan, nonprofit coalition of nine national professional organizations. Its purpose is to advance the health education profession and to mobilize resources for the expansion and improvement of health education through its member organizations.

Web Site: http://www.hsc.usf.edu/CFH/cnheo

Community Campus Partnership for Health (CCPH)

CCPH is a nonprofit organization whose focus is to promote health by creating partnerships between higher institutions of learning and their local communities. Health promotion is accomplished through service-learning projects, community service, community-based research, and other strategies that might be used by the partnerships to improve the health of communities.

Address: 3333 California Street, Suite 410, San Francisco, CA 94118

Web Site: http://www.futurehealth.ucsf.edu/ccph.html

Council on Education for Public Health (CEPH)

CEPH is the national accreditation body for schools of public health and certain graduate public health education programs offered in education settings other than schools of public health. It is the agency recognized by the U.S. Department of Education for this accreditation function.

CEPH aims at promoting quality in education for public health through a continuing process of self-evaluation by the schools and programs that seek accreditation, assuring the public that institutions offering accredited graduate instruction in public health meet standards essential for conducting such programs, and encouraging improvement in the quality of education for public health through periodic review, research, publication, and consultation. The council also establishes its own accreditation policies, procedures, and fees for consultation and accreditation.

Address: 800 I Street, N.W., Suite 202, Washington, DC 20001

Web Site: http://www.ceph.org

Department of Health and Human Services (HHS)

HHS is the principal agency of the United States government for protecting human health. Its programs cover issues relating to services for older Americans, the prevention of domestic violence and child abuse, ensuring that food and medicines are safe, immunizations and the prevention of infectious disease outbreaks, services to low-income families, and many other health-related concerns, including research in medical and social science. It is the largest grant-making agency in the federal government. Operating divisions of HHS include the Food and Drug Administration (FDA), Indian Health Services (IHS), Substance Abuse and Mental Health Services (SAMHS), and Health Resources and Services Administration (HRSA).

Web Site: http://www.hhs.gov

Directors of Health Promotion and Education (DHPE)

DHPE is concerned with developing policies and resources and conducting community-based programs in health promotion and education to prevent disease. It aims at creating public awareness of the need for health promotion, health education, and disease prevention and provides opportunities for continuing education in the fields of health promotion and health education to enhance professional practice. DHPE consists of fifty-five directors of health education and health promotion in the United States and its territories, including the Indian Health Service.

Address: 1101 Fifteenth Street, N.W., Suite 601, Washington, DC 20005

Web Site: http://www.dhpe.org

Food and Drug Administration (FDA)

FDA is a regulatory agency within the U.S. Department of Health and Human Services whose mission is the responsibility of protecting the health of the public by ensuring the safety, efficacy, and security of human and veterinary drugs, biological products, medical devices, the nation's food supply, cosmetics, and products that emit radiation. FDA is also responsible for advancing the public's health by advancing innovations that make medicines and foods more effective, safer, and more affordable and by helping the public get accurate, science-based information needed to use medicines and foods to improve their health.

Web Site: http://www.fda.org

Health Resources and Services Administration (HRSA)

HRSA, an agency of the U. S. Department of Health and Human Services, exists to improve and expand access to quality health care for all Americans, thus eliminating barriers to health care and health disparities.

Address: 5600 Fishers Lane, Rockville, MD 20857

Web Site: http://www.hrsa.gov

International Health Foundation (IHF)

The International Health Foundation, founded in 1969, is a nonprofit organization based in Geneva, Switzerland (with a main office in the

Netherlands), dedicated to advancing the health of humankind by defining human mental, physical, and social problems and contributing to their solutions. IHF promotes research and education, conducts and publishes health-related studies, and publishes a quarterly information bulletin.

Address: Europalaan 506, NL-3526 KS Utrecht, Netherlands

Web Site: http://www.ihf.nl

International Planned Parenthood Federation (IPPF)

IPPF is a nongovernmental, independent association that works to initiate and support family planning services, develop resources, and stimulate research. IPPF currently links national autonomous Family Planning Associations in over 180 countries globally and is committed to promoting the right and freedom of women to decide on the number and spacing of their children. The federation provides several publications, including a bimonthly medical bulletin.

Address: Regent's College, Inner Circle, Regent's Park, London NW1 4NS, United Kingdom

Web Site: http://www.ippf.org

International Society on Hypertension in Blacks (ISHIB)

ISHIB is a nonprofit organization dedicated to improving the health and life expectancy of ethnic populations in the United States and around the world. The organization was founded in Atlanta, Georgia, in 1986 to respond to the problem of high blood pressure among African Americans and has since broadened its mission to include the total spectrum of ethnicity and disease.

ISHIB aims at stimulating research and clinical investigation; disseminating scientific findings to aid in the understanding of differences in obesity, hypertension, and other health issues among ethnic groups; promoting public awareness of the harmful effects of hypertension, especially among African Americans; educating the public on ways to prevent the complications of hypertension; and developing health-related programs to improve the quality of life and health expectancy in ethnic minority populations worldwide.

ISHIB sponsors yearly international conferences at different geographical locations, attracting people in the medical and health care professions from throughout the world who want to learn at first hand the latest in research and clinical practice.

ISHIB publishes a newsletter, as well as a quarterly journal, *Ethnicity and Disease.*

Address: 2045 Manchester Street N.E., Atlanta, GA 30324

Web Site: http://www.ishib.org

International Union for Health Promotion and Education (IUHPE)

IUHPE is an international professional organization committed to advancing public health and the development of health promotion and education around the world. Formerly the International Union for Health Education (IUHE), it now includes health promotion.

IUHPE has constituent, institutional, and individual memberships and works in cooperation with the World Health Organization (WHO), the United Nations Educational, Scientific and Cultural Organization (UNESCO), and the United Nations International Children's Emergency Fund (UNICEF).

IUHPE publishes the journal *Promotion and Education,* an international quarterly journal, and *NARO News.*

Address: 42 Boulevard de la Libération, F-93203 Saint-Denis Cedex, France

Web Site: http://www.iuhpe.org

National Association of Community Health Centers (NACHC)

NACHC is the leading organization representing the nation's network of health centers. It provides services including technical assistance to support health centers in their provision of health services, particularly to the poor and underserved in their community. It is within their mission to advance high-quality, comprehensive health care and making it easily accessible to all underserved groups. NACHC members are kept informed about health care policies and new information on primary health care. In addition, they are provided with educational tools to assist in program development in an effort to eliminate health disparities in populations and improve health outcomes.

Address: 7200 Wisconsin Avenue, Suite 210, Bethesda, MD 20814

Web Site: http://www.nachc.com

National Association of County and City Health Officials (NACCHO)

NACCHO is the national nonprofit organization that represents local government public health agencies, including tribal public health agencies. The organization is involved in providing education, information, research, and technical assistance to health departments.

Address: 1100 Seventeenth Street, N.W., Washington, DC 20036

Web Site: http://www.naccho.org

National Association of Senior Health Professionals (NASHP)

NASHP is a new Web-based membership organization specifically designed to address the unique needs and special interests of professionals in the rapidly growing field of senior health. Membership is open to any professional who works with older adults in the public, private, and nonprofit sectors, including hospital-based senior membership program directors, health educators, health promotion staff, activity professionals, and fitness program and health club staff. Members are provided with instant access to important information related to the association and its goals.

Address: 1850 West Winchester Road, Suite 213, Libertyville, IL 60048

Web Site: http://seniorprograms.com

National Cancer Institute (NCI)

NCI is a constituent of the National Institutes of Health and is the lead agency for cancer research and dissemination of cancer information. It is responsible for coordinating research projects at academic and medical institutions and in industry both domestically and abroad and provides funding through grants for fellowships, research, and training in the prevention, control, and treatment of cancer.

Web Site: http://www.nci.nih.gov

National Center for Complementary and Alternative Medicine (NCCAM)

Established by Congress in 1998, NCCAM is one of the institutes of the National Institutes of Health. Its mission is to explore complementary and alternative health care practices through scientific research and dissemination of research findings to the public. NCCAM is also involved in providing grants for training and career development for researchers and operates a clearinghouse of information for public access.

Address: National Institutes of Health, Bethesda, MD 20892

Web Site: http://nccam.nih.gov

National Center for Health Education

The National Center for Health Education is an independent nonprofit organization established as the lead agency for lifelong comprehensive health education in the United States. Its aim is to provide information exchange, technical assistance, research, and evaluation for improving the health of Americans. The center is also concerned with advocacy and brings together members of diverse groups to discuss issues related to health and health education in an effort to improve health.

Web Site: http://www.nche.org

National Commission for Health Education Credentialing (NCHEC)

NCHEC is the official organization responsible for establishing, implementing, and maintaining a certification process for health education specialists through professional preparation and professional development. Its mission is to improve the quality of health education practice and to ensure continual updating of skills and knowledge.

This organization was established in 1988 and became incorporated as a nonprofit, tax-exempt organization with an elected board of directors. In the early years, experienced health educators were permitted to apply for charter certification, but since 1990, individuals must become certified by passing an examination. Recertification is made available every five years based on continuing-education criteria.

Address: 944 Marcon Boulevard, Suite 310, Allentown, PA 18109

Web Site: http://www.nchec.org

National Council on the Aging (NCOA)

NCOA is the nation's first association of organizations and professionals dedicated to promoting the dignity, self-determination, well-being, and contributions of older persons. Founded in 1950, NCOA is a private, non-profit association consisting of individuals and organizations, including senior centers, adult day service centers, area agencies on aging, employment services, congregate meal sites, faith congregations, health centers, and senior housing.

NCOA is also part of a network of more than seventeen thousand organizations and individuals, including professionals, volunteers, service providers, consumer groups, businesses, government agencies, religious groups, and voluntary organizations, and is a national voice and powerful advocate for public policies, societal attitudes, and business practices that promote vital aging. NCOA often leads campaigns to preserve funding for the Older Americans Act and other government programs that benefit seniors and their families.

Address: 300 D Street, S.W., Suite 801, Washington, DC 20024

Web Site: http://www.ncoa.org

National Environmental Health Association (NEHA)

NEHA originated in California in the late 1930s to establish a standard for environmental health. This has become the credentialing examination now known as the Registered Environmental Health Specialist/Registered Sanitarian. The association now administers seven credential programs. One of the purposes of the association is to promote cooperation among environmental health professionals to assist in resolving global environmental health concerns.

Address: 720 South Colorado Boulevard, South Tower, Suite 970, Denver, CO 80246

Web Site: http://www.neha.org

National Health Information Center (NHIC)

NHIC is a branch of the Office of Disease Prevention and Health Promotion in the U. S. Department of Health and Human Services, designed as a referral service center to put people with health questions in touch with specific organizations that are able to best answer their questions.

Web Site: http://www.health.gov/nhic

National Heart, Lung, and Blood Institute (NHLBI)

NHLBI is one of the constituents of the National Institutes of Health, established to provide leadership in programs related to diseases of the heart, lungs, and blood as well as sleep disorders. NHLBI conducts and supports research and demonstration projects in all aspects of heart, blood, and lung disorders. It also operates an information center to disseminate information, including relevant publications on matters of the heart, lungs, and blood.

Address: Building 31, Room 5A52, 31 Center Drive, MSC 2486, Bethesda, MD 20892

Web Site: http://www.nhlbi.nih.gov

National Institute for Occupational Safety and Health (NIOSH)

NIOSH is the federal agency that conducts research and makes recommendation for preventing injury and illness at the worksite. NIOSH is housed in the U.S. Department of Health and Human Services, headquartered in Washington, D.C., and is part of the Centers for Disease Control and Prevention (CDC). The organization also focuses on education and training in occupational health and safety and provides national leadership in the prevention of occupational injuries for all employees in the workplace.

Web Site: http://www.cdc.gov/niosh

National Institute of Mental Health (NIMH)

NIMH is the largest scientific institute in the world with a primary focus on mental disorders. The institute directs federal efforts to promote mental health, prevent and treat brain disorders and mental illness, and rehabilitate those who suffer from mental conditions.

NIMH conducts and supports research on the biological, psychological, behavioral, clinical, and epidemiological aspects of mental health and on disorders of the brain and mind. In addition, it funds the training of researchers, provides professional assistance to the states and community organizations responsible for mental health programs, and disseminates research findings to health care professionals, the media, and the public.

Address: 6001 Executive Boulevard, Room 8184, Bethesda, MD 20892

Web Site: http://www.nimh.nih.gov

National Institute on Alcohol Abuse and Alcoholism (NIAAA)

NIAAA leads the federal government's efforts to reduce the enormous health, social, and economic consequences of alcohol abuse and alcoholism.

NIAAA operates a research program encompassing a wide range of research in the biomedical and behavioral sciences to include health risks and benefits, prevention, and treatment.

NIAAA supports intramural research facilities, promotes a variety of research efforts, and fosters the development of effective treatment and prevention through the circulation of research findings to health care providers and professionals. The institute has also expanded research on public policy issues such as alcohol taxation, alcohol consumption, warning labels, and drinking-and-driving laws to provide a scientific basis for the development and assessment of public policy.

Address: 6000 Executive Boulevard, Bethesda, MD 20892

Web Site: http://www.niaaa.nih.gov

National Institute on Drug Abuse (NIDA)

NIDA, established in 1974, is the leading federal agency for research on the incidence and prevalence of drug abuse, its causes and consequences, and improved methods of prevention and treatment of drug abuse, with the intention of increasing knowledge and solving problems associated with drug abuse and improving understanding of the effects of drugs.

NIDA supports research on effective prevention and treatment of drug abuse and on the role of drug abuse as a factor in the spread of AIDS. Research findings are usually presented in NIDA research monographs, available from the U.S. Department of Health and Human Services.

Address: 6000 Executive Boulevard, Room 5213, Bethesda, MD 20892

Web Site: http://www.drugabuse.gov

National Institutes of Health (NIH)

NIH started in the late 1880s and is currently the leading federal agency in health research within the U.S. Department of Health and Human Services.

Headquartered in Bethesda, Maryland, "NIH is the steward of medical and behavioral research for the Nation. Its mission is science in pursuit of fundamental knowledge about the nature and behavior of living systems and the application of that knowledge to extend healthy life and reduce the burdens of illness and disability. The goals of the agency are as follows: (1) foster fundamental creative discoveries, innovative research strategies, and their applications as a basis to advance significantly the Nation's capacity to protect and improve health; (2) develop, maintain, and renew scientific human and physical resources that will assure the Nation's capability to prevent disease; (3) expand the knowledge base in medical and associated sciences in order to enhance the Nation's economic well-being and ensure a continued high return on the public investment in research; and (4) exemplify and promote the highest level of scientific integrity, public accountability, and social responsibility in the conduct of science" (National Institutes of Health, 2003).

Web Site: http://www.nih.gov

National Women's Health Information Center

The National Women's Health Information Center is a federal government source for women's health information, maintaining a Web site and a toll-free call center. It was created to provide free, reliable health information for women everywhere.

Call Center: (800) 994-9662; TDD (888) 220-5446 (both toll-free)

Web Site: http://www.4woman.gov

Occupational Safety and Health Administration (OSHA)

OSHA is a federal agency responsible for injury prevention and health protection of workers or employees. It establishes standards and enforces those standards. OSHA also provides technical assistance and training as well as consultation to agencies and organizations and inspects sites to ensure that standards are followed in an effort to reduce occupational hazards and promote safety at work for all workers.

Web Site: http://www.osha.gov

Planned Parenthood Federation of America

Planned Parenthood is the world's largest and most trusted voluntary reproductive health care organization. Founded by Margaret Sanger in 1916 as America's first birth control clinic, Planned Parenthood believes in everyone's right to choose when or whether to have a child, that every child should be wanted and loved, and that women should be in charge of their own destinies. There are a number of branches of this organization in several states.

Address: 1780 Massachusetts Avenue, N.W., Washington, DC 20036

Public Health electronic Library (PHeL)

The Public Health electronic Library is a national "one-stop shop" for all information relating to public health. It aims to provide knowledge and know-how to promote health, prevent disease, and reduce health inequities. Its primary audience is professionals in the public health community. PHeL is a specialist library of the National electronic Library for Health.

Web Site: http://www.phel.gov.uk

Public Health Foundation (PHF)

PHF is a national, private, nonprofit organization dedicated to achieving healthy communities through research, training, and technical assistance. PHF assists health agencies and other community health system organizations by providing objective information in areas such as health improvement planning, understanding and using data, and improving performance.

Address: 1220 L Street, N.W., Suite 350, Washington, DC 20005

Web Site: http://www.phf.org

Public Health Institute (PHI)

PHI, founded in 1964, is an independent, nonprofit organization dedicated to promoting health and quality of life for people throughout California, across the nation, and worldwide. PHI promotes and sustains independent, innovative research, training, and demonstration programs, many in collaboration with the private health care system and community-based organizations.

PHI also serves as a partner with government to support its role in assessment, policy development, and assurance. The quality programs and projects of PHI improve the health of people and communities and inform the development of public policy. The institute is a resource for researchers and professionals who view the social, environmental, economic, and demographic changes in our communities in terms of the impact on health.

Address: 555 Twelfth Street, 10th Floor, Oakland, CA 94607

Web Site: http://www.phi.org

Society for Behavioral Medicine (SBM)

SBM aims at fostering the development and application of knowledge concerning the interrelationships of health, illness, and behavior. It is concerned with developing and integrating knowledge and techniques from behavioral, psychological, and biomedical sciences, through research and practice, in order to better understand health and illness and to influence health care.

Address: 7600 Terrace Avenue, Suite 203, Middleton, WI 53562

Web Site: http://www.sbm.org

Society for Public Health Education (SOPHE)

SOPHE is a national professional service organization, formed in 1950, to promote, encourage, and contribute to the health of all people by stimulating research, developing criteria for professional preparation, elevating performance standards for the practice of health education, promoting networking among health education professionals and public health students, and advocating policy and legislation affecting health education and health promotion.

SOPHE is the only professional organization devoted exclusively to public health education and health promotion. The organization publishes the journals *Health Education Quarterly* and *Health Promotion Practice* and a quarterly newsletter, *News and Views*.

SOPHE sponsors annual and midyear scientific conferences and offers continuing education for professional development of its Certified Health Education Specialists (CHES) members. SOPHE also works with advisory boards and coalitions at the national, state, and local levels to influence health promotion practice and policy decisions. It serves to stimulate peer exchange through its annual membership directory and supports ethical health education research by promoting the SOPHE Code of Ethics.

SOPHE recognizes professional excellence and leadership through Distinguished Fellow, Student Paper, and Program Excellence Awards. The society has many chapters in many states.

Address: 750 First Street, N.E., Suite 910, Washington, DC 20002

Web Site: http://www.sophe.org

Substance Abuse and Mental Health Services Administration (SAMHSA)

SAMHSA is the leading federal agency responsible for improving prevention services for substance abuse and mental illnesses. It was established as an agency of the U.S. Department of Health and Human Services (HHS) by an act of Congress in 1992. "With the stroke of a pen, an agency, separate and distinct from the National Institutes of Health or any other agency within the HHS, was created to focus attention, programs, and funding on improving the lives of people with or at risk for mental and substance abuse disorders" (SAMHSA, 2003).

To promote accountability, enhance capacity, and ensure effectiveness, "SAMHSA tracks national trends, establishes measurement and reporting systems, develops and promotes standards to monitor service systems, and works to achieve excellence in management practices in mental health services, addiction treatment, and substance abuse prevention; assessing resources, supporting systems of community-based care, improving service financing and organization, and promoting a strong, well-educated workforce, SAMHSA enhances the Nation's capacity to serve people with or at risk of mental and substance abuse disorders. The Agency also helps assure service effectiveness through the continuous improvement of services and workforce by assessing service delivery practices, identifying and promoting evidence-based approaches to care, implementing and evaluating innovative services, and providing workforce skills training" (SAMHSA, 2003).

Web Site: http://www.samhsa.gov

United Nations International Children's Emergency Fund (UNICEF)

UNICEF, also known as the United Nations Children's Fund, was established after World War II to assist children in war-torn Europe, mainly through the distribution of powdered milk from the United States. As conditions improved, attention expanded from Europe to needy children throughout the world.

UNICEF instituted programs to control communicable diseases in children, provide clean drinking water, protect children's rights, and promote improved child survival, nutrition, health care, and education to improve the health of children globally.

UNICEF was a cosponsor of the Alma Ata conference in 1978 on primary health care (see *Alma Ata Declaration* in Part One). Funding is through contributions, sale of greeting cards, monies from government and nongovernmental organizations, and other sources (Basch, 1990).

Address: 3 United Nations Plaza, New York, NY 10017

Web Site: http://www.unicef.org

United States Environmental Protection Agency (EPA)

EPA, formed in 1970, is an independent agency of the United States government. It is the primary federal agency charged with protecting human health and safeguarding the natural environment—air, water, and land systems on which life depends.

EPA has been working for a cleaner, healthier environment for the American people. It strives to formulate and implement actions to lead to a compatible balance between human activities and the ability of natural systems to support and nurture life and is responsible for ensuring health and environmental protection. EPA leads the nation's environmental science, research, education, and assessment efforts and publishes a quarterly journal.

Address: 1200 Pennsylvania Avenue, N.W., Washington, DC 20460

Web Site: http://www.epa.gov

Wellness Councils of America (WELCOA)

Based in Omaha, Nebraska, WELCOA was founded in 1987 as a national nonprofit membership organization dedicated to promoting healthier lifestyles for all Americans through health promotion initiatives at the worksite. WELCOA serves as an umbrella, linking communities and coalitions together into a supportive network that includes locally affiliated Wellness Councils, Well City initiatives, Well Workplaces, and individual and corporate members throughout the United States.

In addition to helping organizations build structurally sound wellness programs, WELCOA serves as a national clearinghouse and information center on worksite wellness and responds to requests for information and materials by publishing a number of sourcebooks, a monthly newsletter, and brochures and conducting numerous training seminars.

Address: 9802 Nicholas Street, Suite 315, Omaha, NE 68114

Web Site: http://www.welcoa.org

World Health Organization (WHO)

WHO is an agency of the United Nations that serves as the premier organization in the field of health worldwide. It was established on April 7, 1948, a day annually commemorated as World Health Day. Intended to assist people in attaining the best possible health, WHO is financed by dues from member countries, voluntary funds, and contributions from several sources.

Headquartered in Geneva, Switzerland, with regional headquarters in Europe, the eastern Mediterranean, Africa, Southeast Asia, the western Pacific, and the Americas and collaborating centers and offices in many countries, WHO provides services to governments and central technical services such as information on health aspects of travel and commerce, international standardization of vaccines and pharmaceuticals, and literature disseminating knowledge on world health problems. WHO is committed to major policy decisions affecting the health of people globally, training health personnel, providing services to governments as requested, and assisting governments in reviewing and evaluating health needs and resources.

Address: 525 Twenty-Third Street, N.W., Washington, DC 20037

REFERENCES

Ajzen, I. (1991). The theory of planned behavior. *Organizational Behavior and Human Decision Processes, 50*(2), 179–211.

Anderson, L. A., De Vellis, R. F., Sharpe, P. A., & Marcoux, B. (1994). Multidimensional health locus of control scales: Do they measure expectancies about control or desires for control? *Health Education Research, 9*(1), 145–151.

Anderson, L. W., & Krathwohl, D. (Eds.). (2001). *A taxonomy for learning, teaching, and assessing.* New York: Longman.

Aronson, E. (1992). The return of the repressed: Dissonance theory makes a comeback. *Psychological Inquiry, 3*(4), 303–311.

Association for the Advancement of Health Education (AAHE). (1994). Code of ethics for health educators. *Journal of Health Education, 25*(4), 197–200.

Austin, J. E. (2000). *The collaborative challenge: How nonprofits and businesses succeed through strategic alliances.* San Francisco: Jossey-Bass.

Backett, K., Davison, C., & Mullen, K. (1994). Lay evaluation of health and healthy lifestyles: Evidence from three studies. *British Journal of General Practice, 44*(383), 277–280.

Basch, P. F. (1990). *Textbook of international health.* New York: Oxford University Press.

Baulcomb, J. S. (2003). Management of change through force field analysis. *Journal of Nursing Management, 11*(4), 275–280.

Bedworth, A. E., & Bedworth, D. A. (1992). *The profession and practice of health education.* Dubuque, IA: Brown & Benchmark.

Belzer, E. G., & McIntyre, L. (1994). A model for coordinating school health promotion programs. *Journal of School Health, 64*(5), 196–200.

Benenson, A. (1990). *Control of communicable diseases in man.* Washington, DC: American Public Health Association.

Benson, S. G., & Dundis, S. P. (2003). Understanding and motivating health care employees: Integrating Maslow's hierarchy of needs, training, and technology. *Journal of Nursing Management, 11*(5), 315–320.

Bodenheimer, T. S., & Grumbach, K. (2002). *Understanding health policy: A clinical approach* (3rd ed.). New York: Lange Medical Books/McGraw-Hill.

Bond, M. J., & Clark, M. S. (2002). A comparison of alternative indices of abnormal illness behavior derived from the Illness Behavior Questionnaire. *Psychology, Health and Medicine, 7*(2), 203–213.

Bracht, N. (Ed.). (1990). *Health promotion at the community level.* Newbury Park, CA: Sage.

Brandon, P. (1993). School health services. A dimension of health care reform. *Oregon Nurse, 58*(2), 7–8.

Breckon, D. J. (1997). *Managing health promotion programs: Leadership skills for the 21st century.* Gaithersburg, MD: Aspen.

Breckon, D. J., Harvey, J. R., & Lancaster, R. B. (1994). *Community health education: Settings, roles, and skills for the 21st century* (3rd ed.). Gaithersburg, MD: Aspen.

Brindis, C. (1993). Health policy reform and comprehensive school health education: The need for an effective partnership. *Journal of School Health, 63*(1), 33–37.

Bryant, C., & Gulitz, E. (1993). Focus group discussions: An application to teaching. *Journal of Health Education, 24*(3), 188–189.

Bunton, R., & Macdonald, G. (1992). *Health promotion: Disciplines and diversity.* New York: Routledge, Chapman, & Hall.

Butler, J. T. (2000). *Principles of health promotion and education* (3rd ed.). Belmont, CA: Wadsworth.

Carey, V., Chapman, S., & Gaffney, D. (1994). Children's lives and garden aesthetics? A case study in public health advocacy. *Australian Journal of Public Health, 18*(1), 25–32.

Carkenord, D. M., & Bullington, J. (1993). Bringing cognitive dissonance to the classroom. *Teaching of Psychology, 20*(1), 41–43.

Cartwright, S. (1993). Cooperative learning can occur in any kind of program. *Young Children, 48*(2), 12–14.

Catania, J. A., & Dolcini, M. (2002). A commentary on Sallies, Owen, and Fotheringham's perspective on "behavioral epidemiology": A systematic framework to classify phases of research on health promotion and disease prevention. *Annals of Behavioral Medicine, 24*(2), 78.

Chenoweth, D. H. (1991). *Planning health promotion at the worksite* (2nd ed.). Dubuque, IA: Brown & Benchmark.

Chiang, L., Huang, J., & Lu, C. (2003). Educational diagnosis of self-management behaviors of parents with asthmatic children by triangulation based on PRECEDE-PROCEED model in Taiwan. *Patient Education and Counseling, 49*(1), 19–25.

Chin, J. (2002). *Control of communicable diseases manual* (17th ed). Washington, DC: American Public Health Association.

Clark, J. K., Ogletree, R. J., McKenzie, J. F., Dennis, D., & Chamness, B. E. (2002). An assessment of health education responsibilities and competencies addressed in continuing education contact hour articles. *American Journal of Health Education, 33*(4), 234–239.

Cleary, M. J. (1993a). Credentialing and vendorship: Are we ready? *Journal of Health Education, 24*(5), 285–287.

Cleary, M. J. (1993b). Using portfolios to assess student performance in school health education. *Journal of School Health, 63*(9), 377–381.

Cooper, J. (1992). Dissonance and the return of the self-concept. *Psychological Inquiry, 3*(4), 320–323.

Cormier, R. M. (2002). Predicting treatment outcome in chemically dependent women: A test of Marlatt and Gordon's relapse model. *Dissertation Abstracts International: The Sciences and Engineering, 62*(10-B), 4777.

Cornacchia, H. J., Olsen, H. K., & Nickerson, C. J. (1991). *Health in elementary schools.* Saint Louis, MO: Mosby Year Book.

Cowley, S. (1994). Collaboration in health care: The education link. *Health Visit, 67*(1), 13–15.

Crane, C., & Martin, M. (2002). Adult illness behavior: The impact of childhood experience. *Personality and Individual Differences, 32*(5), 785–798.

Creswell, J. W. (1994). *Research design: Qualitative and quantitative approaches.* Thousand Oaks, CA: Sage.

DesCamp, K. D., & Thomas, C. C. (1993). Buffering nursing stress through play at work. *Western Journal of Nursing Research, 15*(5), 619–627.

Diamond, G. A. (1992). Field theory and rational choice: A Lewinian approach to modeling motivation. *Journal of Social Issues, 48*(2), 79–94.

Di Clemente, C. C., & Hughes, S. O. (1990). Stages of change profiles in outpatient alcoholism treatment. *Journal of Substance Abuse, 2*, 217–237.

Di Clemente, C. C., et al. (1991). The process of smoking cessation: An analysis of precontemplation, contemplation, and preparation stages of change. *Journal of Consulting and Clinical Psychology, 59*(2), 295–304.

Doll, J., & Ajzen, I. (1992). Accessibility and stability of predictors in the theory of planned behavior. *Journal of Personality and Social Psychology, 63*(5), 754–765.

Ellis, G. A., Reed, D. F., & Scheider, H. (1995). Mobilizing a low-income African American community around tobacco control: A force field analysis. *Health Education Quarterly, 22*(4), 443–457.

Emlet, C. A., & Hall, A. M. (1991). Integrating the community into geriatric case management: Public health interventions. *Gerontologist, 31*(4), 556–560.

Farley, S. D., & Stasson, M. F. (2003). Relative influences of affect and cognition on behavior: Are feelings or beliefs more related to blood donation intentions? *Experimental Psychology, 50*(1), 55–62.

Fenlason, K. J., & Beehr, T. A. (1994). Social support and occupational stress: Effects of talking to others. *Journal of Organizational Behavior, 15*(2), 157–175.

Fetterman, D. M. (2002). Empowerment evaluation building communities of practice and a culture of learning. *American Journal of Community Psychology, 30*(1), 89–102.

Finfgeld, D. L., Wongvatunyu, S., Conn, V. S., Grando, V. T., & Russell, C. L. (2003). Health belief model and reversal therapy: A comparative analysis. *Journal of Advanced Nursing, 43*(3), 288.

Foreyt, J. P., Goodrick, G. K., Reeves, R. S., & Raynaud, A. S. (1993). Response of free-living adults to behavioral treatment of obesity: Attrition and compliance to exercise. *Behavior Therapy, 24*(4), 659–669.

Gibbie, K., Rosenstock, L., & Hernandez, L. (Eds.). (2003). *Who will keep the public healthy in the 21st century?* Washington, DC: National Academy Press.

Girvan, J. T., Hamburg, M. V., & Miner, K. R. (1993). Credentialing the health education profession. *Journal of Health Education, 24*(5), 260.

Glantz, K., Lewis, F. M., & Rimer, B. K. (1990). *Health behavior and health education: Theory, research, and practice.* San Francisco: Jossey-Bass.

Gonder-Frederick, L. A., Cox, D. J., & Ritterband, L. M. (2002). Diabetes and behavioral medicine: The second decade. *Journal of Consulting and Clinical Psychology, 70*(3), 611–625.

Goodman, R. M., et al. (1998). Identifying and defining the dimensions of community capacity to provide a basis for measurement. *Health Education and Behavior, 25*(3), 258–278.

Goodman, S. H., Cooley, E., Sewell, D. R., & Leavitt, N. (1994). Locus of control and self-esteem in depressed, low-income African American women. *Community Mental Health Journal, 30*(3), 259–269.

Graeff, J. A., Elder, T. P., & Mills-Booth, E. (1993). *Communication for health and behavior change: A developing-country perspective.* San Francisco: Jossey-Bass.

Green, L. W., & Kreuter, M. W. (1991). *Health promotion planning: An educational and environmental approach.* Mountain View, CA: Mayfield.

Green, L. W., & Kreuter, M. W. (1999). *Health promotion planning: An educational and ecological approach* (3rd ed.). Mountain View, CA: Mayfield.

Greenberg, J. S. (1992). *Health education.* Dubuque, IA: Brown.

Grilo, C. M., & Shiffman, S. (1994). Longitudinal investigation of the abstinence violation effect in binge eaters. *Journal of Consulting and Clinical Psychology, 62*(3), 611–619.

Grover, S. A., Gray, D. K., Joseph, L., Abrahamowicz, M., & Coupal, L. (1994). Life expectancy following dietary modification or smoking cessation: Estimating the benefits of a prudent lifestyle. *Archives of Internal Medicine, 154*(15), 1697–1704.

Grunbaum, J. A., & Basen-Engquist, K. (1993). Comparison of health risk behaviors between students in a regular high school and students in an alternative high school. *Journal of School Health, 63*(10), 421–425.

Hall, S. M., Munoz, R. F., & Reus, V. I. (1994). Cognitive-behavioral intervention increases abstinence rates for depressive-history smokers. *Journal of Consulting and Clinical Psychology, 62*(1), 141–146.

Hamburg, M. V. (1993). Perspectives on teaching comprehensive school health. *Preventive Medicine, 22*(4), 533–543.

Handler, A., Schieve, L. A., Ippoliti, P., Gordon, A. K., & Turnock, B. J. (1994). Building bridges between schools of public health and public health practice. *American Journal of Public Health, 84*(7), 1077–1080.

Harrington, C., & Estes, C. L. (2001). *Health policy: Crisis and reform in the U.S. health care delivery system.* Sudbury, MA: Jones & Bartlett.

Hermann, C., Blanchard, E. B., & Flor, H. (1997). Biofeedback treatment for pediatric migraine: Prediction of treatment outcome. *Journal of Consulting and Clinical Psychology, 65*(4), 611–616.

Himsl, R., & Lambert, E. (1993). Signs of learning in the affective domain. *Alberta Journal of Educational Research, 39*(2), 257–273.

Howze, E. H., & Redman, L. J. (1992). The uses of theory in health advocacy: Policies and programs. *Health Education Quarterly, 19*(3), 369–383.

Huber, G. L. (2003). Processes of decision-making in small learning groups. *Learning and Instruction, 13*(3), 255–269.

Huff, R. M., & Kline, M. V. (1999). *Promoting health in multicultural populations: A handbook for practitioners.* Thousand Oaks, CA: Sage.

Hunt, M. K., et al. (1990). Pawtucket heart health program point-of-purchase nutrition education program in supermarkets. *American Journal of Public Health, 80*(6), 730–732.

Hunter, L. (2004). Life and its molecules: A brief introduction. *AL Magazine, 25*(1), 9–22.

Israel, B. A., Checkoway, B., Schulz, A., & Zimmerman, M. (1994). Health education and community empowerment: Conceptualizing and measuring perceptions of individual, organizational, and community control. *Health Education Quarterly, 21*(2), 149–170.

James, L. D., Thorn, B. E., & Williams, D. A. (1993). Goal specification in cognitive-behavioral therapy for chronic headache pain. *Behavior Therapy, 24*(2), 305–320.

Kaplan, R. M. (1990). Behavior as the central outcome in health care. *American Psychologist, 45*(11), 1211–1220.

Kaplan, R. M., Sallis, J. F., Jr., & Patterson, T. L. (1993). *Health and human behavior.* San Francisco: McGraw-Hill.

Keefe, F. J., Buffington, A. I., Studts, J. L., & Rumble, M. E. (2002). Behavioral medicine: 2002 and beyond. *Journal of Consulting and Clinical Psychology, 70*(3), 852–856.

King, C. K., Glass, R., Bresee, J. S., & Duggan, C. (2003). Managing acute gastroenteritis among children, oral rehydration maintenance, and nutritional therapy. *Morbidity and Mortality Weekly Report, 52*(Suppl. RR-16), 1–16.

Knutsen, S. F. (1994). Lifestyle and the use of health services. *American Journal of Clinical Nutrition, 59*(Suppl. 5), 1171S–1175S.

Kotler, P., Roberto, N., & Lee, N. (2002). *Social Marketing: Improving the Quality of Life.* (2nd ed.). Thousand Oaks, CA: Sage.

Laberge, B., Gauthier, J. G., Cote, G., Plamondon, J., & Cormier, H. J. (1993). Cognitive behavioral therapy of panic disorder with secondary major depression: A preliminary investigation. *Journal of Consulting and Clinical Psychology, 61*(6), 1028–1037.

Labonte, R. (1994). Health promotion and empowerment: Reflections on professional practice. *Health Education Quarterly, 21*(2), 253–268.

Lasater, T. M., et al. (1991). Community-based approach to weight loss: The Pawtucket weigh-in. *Addictive Behavior, 16*(3–4), 175–181.

Lester, D. (1990). Maslow's hierarchy of needs and personality. *Personality and Individual Differences, 11*(11), 1187–1188.

Levy, S. R., Baldyga, W., & Jurkowski, J. N. (2003). Developing community health promotion interventions: Selecting partners and fostering collaboration. *Health Promotion Practice, 4*(3), 314–322.

Lim, V. J., Modeste, N. N., & Williams, Y. (2003). Personalized enhancement smoking cessation training program(PEP). *California Journal of Health Promotion, 1*(4), 30–37.

Litwin, M. S. (1995). *How to measure survey reliability and validity.* Thousand Oaks, CA: Sage.

Livingood, W. C., et al. (1993). Credentialing and competition for social jurisdiction. *Journal of Health Education, 24*(5), 282–284.

Lowis, A. (1992). Moving to a community based curriculum. *Occupational Health London, 44*(12), 368.

Lupton, D. (1994). Toward the development of critical health communication praxis. *Health Communication, 6*(1), 55–67.

Luquis, R. R., & Pérez, M. A (2003). Achieving cultural competence: The challenges for health educators. *American Journal of Health Education, 34*(3), 131–140.

Mail, P. D. (1993). A national profile of health educators: Preliminary data from the first cohorts of CHES. *Journal of Health Education, 24*(5), 269–277.

Marcus, B. H., et al. (2000). Physical activity behavior change: Issues in adoption and maintenance. *Health Psychology, 19*(1 Suppl.), 32–41.

Marlatt, G. A., & Gordon, J. R. (Eds.). (1985). *Relapse prevention Maintenance strategies in the treatment of addictive behaviors.* New York: Guilford Press.

Martin, G., & Pear, J. (1992). *Behavior modification.* Englewood Cliffs, NJ: Prentice Hall.

Masalu, J. R., & Åstrøm, A. N. (2003). The use of the theory of planned behavior to explore beliefs about sugar restriction. *American Journal of Health Behavior, 27*(1), 15–24.

McConnell, C. R. (1998). *Case studies in health care supervision.* Gaithersburg, MD: Aspen.

McKenzie, J. F., & Jurs, J. L. (1993). *Planning, implementing, and evaluating health programs.* New York: Macmillan.

McKenzie, J. F., Pinger, R. R., & Kotecki, J. E. (2002). *An introduction to community health* (4th ed.). Boston: Jones & Bartlett.

McMahon, R. C., Schram, L. L., & Davidson, R. S. (1993). Negative life events, social support, and depression in three personality types. *Journal of Personality Disorders, 7*(3), 241–254.

McMaster, C., & Lee, C. (1991). Cognitive dissonance in tobacco smokers. *Addictive Behaviors, 16*(5), 349–353.

Minkler, M., & Wallerstein, N. (2003). *Community-based participatory research for health.* San Francisco: Jossey-Bass.

Modeste, N. N. (1994). Worksite health promotion for women. *Promotion and Education, 1*(1), 29–33.

Moorhead, R. G. (1992). Who do people talk to about healthy lifestyles? A South Australian survey. *Family Practice, 9*(4), 472–475.

Moorman, C. (2002). Consumer health under the scope. *Journal of Consumer Research, 29*(1), 152.

National Institutes of Health, Bioinformatics Definition Committee. (2000, July 17). *NIH working definition of bioinformatics and computational biology.* Retrieved from http://www.bisti.nih.gov/CompuBioDef.pdf.

National Institutes of Health. (2003). *NIH overview and organization.* Retrieved from http://www.bisti.nih.gov/about/NIHoverview.html.

1990 Joint Committee on Health Education Terminology. (1991). Report of the 1990 Joint Committee on Health Education Terminology. *Journal of Public Health Education, 22*(2), 97–107.

Okonski, V. O. (2003). Exercise as a counseling intervention. *Journal of Mental Health Counseling, 25*(1), 45–56.

Ornish, D., et al. (1990). Can lifestyle changes reverse heart disease? The lifestyle heart trial. *Lancet, 336*(8708), 129–133.

Ovrebo, B., Ryan, M., Jackson, K., & Hutchinson, K. (1994). The homeless prenatal program: A model for empowering homeless pregnant women. *Health Education Quarterly, 21*(2), 187–198.

Owen, N., & Crawford, D. (2001). Health promotion: Perspectives on physical activity and weight control. In D. W. Johnston & M. Johnston (Eds.), *Health psychology: Vol. 8. Comprehensive clinical psychology* (pp. 675–689). New York: Pergamon Press.

Parks, G. A., Anderson, B. K., & Marlatt, G. A. (2001). Relapse prevention therapy. In N. Heather, T. J. Peters, & T. Stockwell, T. (Eds.), *International handbook of alcohol dependence and problems* (pp. 575–592). Chichester, England: Wiley.

Powers, B. A., & Knapp, T. (1990). *A dictionary of nursing theory and research.* Newbury Park, CA: Sage.

Pruitt, S. D., Klapow, J. C., Epping-Jordan, J. E., & Dresselhaus, T. R. (1998). Moving behavioral medicine to the front line: A model for the integration of behavioral and medical sciences in primary care. *Professional Psychology: Research and Practice, 29*(3), 230–236.

Quality of life as a new public health measure: Behavioral risk factor surveillance systems, 1993. (1994). *Morbidity and Mortality Weekly Report, 43,* 375–380.

Rajecki, B. W. (1990). *Attitudes.* Sunderland, MA: Sinauer Associates.

Revenson, T. A., & Majerovitz, S. D. (1991). The effects of chronic illness on the spouse: Social resources as stress buffers. *Arthritis Care and Research, 4*(2), 63–72.

Ritchie, J. E. (1994). Education for primary health care: Accommodating the new realities. *World Health Forum, 15*(2), 147–149.

Rodgers, W. M., & Brawley, L. R. (1993). Using both self-efficacy theory and the theory of planned behavior to discriminate adherers and dropouts from structured programs. *Journal of Applied Sport Psychology, 5*(2), 195–206.

Roper, W. L. (1993). Health communication takes on new dimensions at CDC. *Public Health Reports, 108*(2), 179–183.

Rosenstock, I. M. (1991). The Health Belief Model: Explaining health behavior through expectancies. In K. Glantz, F. M. Lewis, & B. K. Rimer (Eds.), *Health behavior and health education: Theory, research, and practice* (pp. 39–62). San Francisco: Jossey-Bass.

Rotter, J. B. (1992). Cognates of personal control: Locus of control, self-efficacy, and explanatory style: Comment. *Applied and Preventive Psychology, 1*(2), 127–129.

Rowitz, L. (2001). *Public health leadership: Putting principles into practice.* Gaithersburg, MD: Aspen.

Rudd, R. E., & Walsh, D. C. (1993). Schools as healthful environments: Prerequisite to comprehensive school health? *Preventive Medicine, 22*(4), 499–506.

Sallis, J. F., Owen, N., & Fotheringham, M. J. (2000). Behavioral epidemiology: A systematic framework to classify phases of research on health promotion and disease prevention. *Annals of Behavioral Medicine, 22*(4), 294–298.

Sarvela, P. D., & McDermott, R. J. (1993). *Health education evaluation and measurement: A practitioner's perspective.* Dubuque, IA: Brown & Benchmark.

Satcher, D., & Bradford, M. T. (2003). Healthy schools, healthy kids. *American School board Journal, 190*(3), 22–25.

Schall, E. (1994). School-based health education: What works? *American Journal of Preventive Medicine, 10*(Suppl. 3), 30–32.

Schiffman, L. G., & Kanuk, L. L. (1991). *Consumer Behavior* (4th ed.). Englewood Cliffs, NJ: Prentice-Hall.

Schwarzer, R., & Renner, B. (2000). Social-cognitive predictors of health behavior: Action self-efficacy and coping self-efficacy. *Health Psychology, 19*(5), 487–495.

Scutchfield, F. D., & Keck, C. W. (2003). *Principles of public health practice* (2nd ed.). Clifton Park, NY: Delmar.

Seaward, B. L. (1994). *Managing stress.* Boston: Jones & Bartlett.

Seffrin, J. (1990). The comprehensive school health curriculum: Closing the gap between state of the art and state of the practice. *Journal of School Health, 60*(4), 151–156.

Shapiro, A. M. (1999). The relevance of hierarchies to learning biology from hypertext. *Journal of Learning Sciences, 8*(2), 215–243.

Shiffman, S., et al. (1996). Progression from a smoking lapse to relapse: Prediction from abstinence violation effects, nicotine dependence, and lapse characteristics. *Journal of Consulting and Clinical Psychology, 64*(5), 993–1002.

Siegel, M., & Doner, L. (1998). *Marketing public health: Strategies to promote social change.* Gaithersburg, MD: Aspen.

Sinha, D. P. (1992). Project lifestyle: Developing positive health lifestyles for school children in Antigua. *Journal of School Health, 62*(10), 449–453.

Slavin, R. E., Hurley, E. A., & Chamberlain, A. (2003). Cooperative learning and achievement: Theory and research. In W. M. Reynolds & G. E. Miller (Eds.), *Handbook of psychology: Educational psychology.* New York: Wiley.

Soriano, F. I. (1995). *Conducting needs assessment: A multidisciplinary approach.* Thousand Oaks, CA: Sage.

Statham, D. (1994). Working together in community care. *Health Visit, 67*(1), 16–18.

Steckler, A., McLeroy, K. R., Goodman, R. M., Bird, S. T., & McCormick, L. (1992). *Toward integrating qualitative and quantitative methods: An introduction.* Health Education Quarterly, *19*(1), 1–8.

Stokols, D. (1992). Establishing and maintaining healthy environments: Toward a social ecology of health promotion. *American Psychologist, 47*(1), 6–22.

Stratton, K., Shetty, P., Wallace, R., & Bondurant, S. (2001). *Clearing the smoke: Assessing the science base for harm reduction.* Washington, DC: Institute of Medicine and National Academy Press.

Strecher, V. J., & Rosenstock, I. M. (1997). The health belief model. In K. Glanz, F. M. Lewis, & B. K. Rimer (Eds.), *Health beliefs and health education: Theory, research, and practice* (pp. 41–59). San Francisco: Jossey-Bass.

Substance Abuse and Mental Health Services Administration. (2003). *The Substance Abuse and Mental Health Services Administration: Promoting a life in the community for everyone.* Retrieved from http://www.samhsa.gov/about/about.html.

Taras, H. L. (1994, Spring). School health clinics. *California Pediatrician,* pp. 31–33.

Tischler, H. L. (1993). *Introduction to sociology.* Fort Worth, TX: Harcourt.

2000 Joint Committee on Health Education Terminology. (2001). Report of the 2000 Joint Committee on Health Education and Promotion Terminology. *Journal of Health Education, 32*(2), 90–103.

Ulbrich, P. M., & Bradsher, J. E. (1993). Perceived support, help seeking, and adaptation to stress among older black and white women living alone. *Journal of Aging and Health, 5*(3), 365–386.

U.S. Department of Health and Human Services. (2000). *Healthy people 2010: Understanding and improving health* (Vols. 1 & 2). Washington, DC: Government Printing Office.

U.S. Public Health Service. (1990). *Healthy people 2000: National health promotion and disease prevention objectives.* Washington, DC: U.S. Department of Health and Human Services.

Valente, T. W. (1993). Diffusion of innovations and policy decision-making. *Journal of Communication, 43*(1), 30–45.

Vlisides, C. E., Eddy, J. P., & Mozie, D. (1994). Stress and stressors: Definition, identification and strategy for higher education constituents. *College Student Journal, 28*(1), 122–124.

Vogt, P. W. (1993). *Dictionary of statistics and methodology.* Newbury Park, CA: Sage.

Wallack, L., Dorfman, L., Jernigan, D., & Themba, D. (1993). *Media advocacy and public health.* Newbury Park, CA: Sage.

Waller, J. V., & Goldman, L. (1993). Bringing comprehensive health education in the New York City public schools: A private-public success story. *Bulletin of the New York Academy of Medicine, 70*(3), 171–187.

Wallerstein, N., & Bernstein, E. (1994). Introduction to community empowerment, participatory education, and health. *Health Education Quarterly, 21*(2), 141–148.

Wankel, L. M., & Mummery, W. K. (1993). Using national survey data incorporating the theory of planned behavior: Implications for social marketing strategies in physical activity. *Journal of Applied Sport Psychology, 5*(2), 158–177.

Watanabe, M. (2004, April 1). Changing of the guard. *Nature,* pp. 584–585.

Whitehead, W. E., (1994). Assessing the effects of stress on physical symptoms. *Health Psychology, 13*(2), 99–102.

Whitfield, K. E., Weidner, G., Clark, R., & Anderson, N. B. (2002). Sociodemographic diversity and behavioral medicine. *Journal of Consulting and Clinical Psychology, 70*(3), 463–481.

Wilson, K. L., & Schuler, K. E. (2002). Coordinating school health programs: Tracing the history of terminology. *Health Education Monograph Series: Student Monographs, 19*(2), 36–39.

Windsor, R., Baranowski, T., Clark, N., & Cutter, G. (1994). *Evaluation of health promotion, health education, and disease prevention programs.* Mountain View, CA: Mayfield.

Wurzbach, M. E. (Ed.). (2002). *Community health education and promotion: A guide to program design and evaluation.* Gaithersburg, MD: Aspen.

Yates, S. (1994). The practice of school nursing: Integration with new models of health service delivery. *Journal of School Nursing, 10*(1), 10–19.

Zimmerman, R. S., & Olson, K. (1994). AIDS-related risk behavior and behavior change in a sexually active, heterosexual sample: A test of three models of prevention. *AIDS Education and Prevention, 6*(3), 189–204.

RECOMMENDED READING

Aday, L. A. (1991). *Designing and conducting health surveys.* San Francisco: Jossey-Bass.

Ahijevych, K., & Bernhard, L. (1994). Health-promoting behaviors of African American women. *Nursing Research, 43*(2), 86–89.

Baker, D., & Klein, R. (1991). Explaining outputs of primary health care: Population and practice factors. *British Medical Journal, 303*(6796), 225–229.

Baronowski, J. (1992–1993). Beliefs as motivational influences at stages in behavior change. *International Quarterly of Community Health Education, 13*(1), 3–29.

Bauman, L. J., & Greenberg Adair, E. G. (1992). The use of ethnographic interviewing to inform questionnaire construction. *Health Education Quarterly, 19*(1), 9–23.

Beilin, L. J. (1990). Diet and lifestyle in hypertension: Changing perspectives. *Cardiovascular Pharmacology, 16*(Suppl. 7), S62–S66.

Birke, S. A., Eldermann, R. T., & Davis, P. E. (1990). An analysis of the abstinence violation effect in a sample of illicit drug users. *British Journal of Addiction, 85*(10), 1299–1307.

Bradley, R. H., et al. (1994). Early indications of resilience and their relation to experiences in the home environments of low birthweight, premature children living in poverty. *Child Development, 65*(2), 346–360.

Breckon, D. J., Harvey, J. R., & Lancaster, R. B. (1994). *Community health education: Settings, roles, and skills for the 21st century* (3rd ed.). Gaithersburg, MD: Aspen.

Brick, P., & Roffman, D. M. (1993). Abstinence, no buts is simplistic. *Educational Leadership, 51*(3), 90–92.

Bruess, C. E. (2003). The importance of health educators as role models. *American Journal of Health Education, 34*(4), 237–239.

Burns, D. D., & Nolen-Hoeksema, S. (1991). Coping styles, homework compliance, and the effectiveness of cognitive-behavioral therapy. *Journal of Consulting and Clinical Psychology, 59*(2), 305–311.

Caira, N. M., et al. (2003). The health educator's role in advocacy and policy: Principles, processes, programs, and partnerships. *Health Promotion Practice, 4*(3), 303–313.

Carkenord, D. M., & Bullington, J. (1993). Bringing cognitive dissonance to the classroom. *Teaching of Psychology, 20*(1), 41–43.

Christianson, J. B., Lurie, N., Finch, M., Moscovice, I. S., & Hartley, D. (1992). Use of community-based mental health programs by HMOs: Evidence from a Medicaid demonstration. *American Journal of Public Health, 82*(6), 790–795.

Clark, N. M., Janz, N. K., Dodge, J. A., & Sharpe, P. A. (1992). Self-regulation of health behavior: The Take PRIDE program. *Health Education Quarterly, 19*(3), 341–354.

Coeling, H. V., & Wilcox, J. R. (1994). Steps to collaboration. *Nursing Administration Quarterly, 18*(4), 44–55.

Conrad, K. M., Riedel, J. E., & Gibbs, J. O. (1990). Effect of worksite health promotion programs on employee absenteeism. A comparative analysis. *American Association of Occupational Health Nurses Journal, 38*(12), 573–580.

Cross, H. D. (1994). An adolescent health and lifestyle guidance system. *Adolescence, 29*(114), 267–277.

Darr, K. (1991). *Ethics in health services management.* Baltimore: Health Professions Press.

Deeds, S. G. (1992). *The health education specialist: Self-study for professional competence.* Los Alamitos, CA: Loose Canon.

Dwyer, T., Viney, R., & Jones, M. (1991). Assessing school health education programs. *International Journal of Technology Assessment and Health Care, 7*(3), 286–295.

Eisen, M., Zellman, G. L., & McAlister, A. L. (1992). A health belief model social learning theory approach to adolescents' fertility control: Findings from a controlled field trial. *Health Education Quarterly, 19*(2), 249–262.

Elliott, C. H., Adams, R. L., & Hodge, G. K. (1992). Cognitive therapy: Possible strategies for optimizing outcome. *Psychiatric Annals, 22*(9), 459–463.

Eng, E., Salmon, M. E., & Mullan, F. (1992). Community empowerment: The critical base for primary health care. *Family and Community Health, 15*(1), 1–12.

Ferguson, E. (1993). Rotter's Locus of Control Scale: A ten-item two-factor model. *Psychological Reports, 73*(3, pt. 2), 1216–1278.

Ferrini, R., Edelstein, S., & Barrett-Connor, E. (1994). The association between health beliefs and health behavior change in older adults. *Preventive Medicine, 23*(1), 1–5.

Fisher, G. L., & Harrison, T. C. (1993). The school counselor's role in relapse prevention. *School Counselor, 41*(2), 120–125.

Fitzpatrick, J. L., & Gerard, K. (1993). Community attitude toward drug use: The need to assess community norms. *International Journal of the Addictions, 28*(10), 947–957.

Flynn, B. C., Ray, D. W., & Rider, M. S. (1994). Empowering communities: Action research. *Health Education Quarterly, 21*(3), 395–405.

172

Fonnebo, V. (1994). The healthy Seventh-Day Adventist lifestyle: What is the Norwegian experience? *American Journal of Clinical Nutrition, 59*(Suppl. 5), 1124S–1129S.

Fowler, B. (1991). A health education program for inner city high school youths: Promoting positive health behaviors through intervention. *Association of Black Nursing Faculty in Higher Education Journal, 2*(3), 53–58.

Freda, M. C., et al. (1990). Lifestyle modification as an intervention for inner city women at high risk for preterm birth. *Journal of Advanced Nursing, 15*(3), 364–372.

French, B. N., Kurczynski, T. W., Weaver, M. T., & Pituch, M. J. (1992). Evaluation of the Health Belief Model and decision making regarding amniocentesis in women of advanced maternal age. *Health Education Quarterly, 19*(2), 177–186.

Friedman, R. A., & Podolny, J. (1992). Differentiation of boundary spanning roles: Labor negotiations and implications for role conflict. *Administrative Science Quarterly, 37*(1), 28–47.

Gallagher, H. G., & Phelan, D. M. (1992). Oral rehydration therapy: A Third World solution applied to intensive care. *Intensive Care Medicine, 18*(1), 53–55.

Garfinkel, A., Allen, L. Q., & Newharth-Pritchett, S. (1993). Foreign language for the gifted: Extending affective dimensions. *Roeper Review, 15*(4), 235–238.

Glanz, K., Lewis, F. M., & Rimer, B. K. (Eds.). (1990). *Health behavior and health education: Theory, research, and practice.* San Francisco: Jossey-Bass.

Gopaldas, T., Gujral, S., Mujoo, R., & Abbi, R. (1991). Child diarrhea: Oral rehydration therapy and rural mothers. *Nutrition, 7*(5), 335–339.

Green, L. W. (1990). *Community health.* Saint Louis, MO: Times Mirror/Mosby.

Grilo, C. M., & Shiffman, S. (1994). Longitudinal investigation of the abstinence violation effect in binge eaters. *Journal of Consulting and Clinical Psychology, 62*(3), 611–619.

Gruder, C. L., et al. (1993). Effects of social support and relapse prevention training as adjuncts to a televised smoking cessation intervention. *Journal of Consulting and Clinical Psychology, 61*(1), 113–120.

Halpern, M. T. (1994). Effects of smoking characteristics on cognitive dissonance in current and former smokers. *Addictive Behaviors, 19*(2), 209–217.

Hochbaum, G. M., Sorenson, J. R., & Lorig, K. (1992). Theory in health education practice. *Health Education Quarterly, 19*(3), 295–313.

Hoppe, M. J., Wells, E. A., Wilsdon, A., Gilmore, M. R., & Morrison, D. M. (1994). Children's knowledge and beliefs about AIDS: Qualitative data from focus group interviews. *Health Education Quarterly, 2*(1), 117–126.

Johnson, A. A., et al. (1994). Selected lifestyle practices in urban African-American women: Relationships to pregnancy outcome, dietary intakes and anthropometric measurements. *Journal of Nutrition, 124*(Suppl. 6), 963S–972S.

Kalnins, I., Mahon, S. M., & Casperson, D. S. (1994). Benefits of collaboration in continuing education: A partnership between a university provider and a nursing specialty organization. *Journal of Continuing Education in Nursing, 25*(4), 148–151.

Kasen, S., Vaughan, R. D., & Walter, H. J. (1992). Self-efficacy for AIDS prevention behaviors among tenth grade students. *Health Education Quarterly, 19*(2), 187–202.

Kashima, Y., Gallois, C., & McCamish, M. (1993). The theory of reasoned action and cooperative behavior: It takes two to use a condom. *British Journal of Social Psychology, 32*(3), 227–239.

Katz, P. P., & Showstack, J. A. (1990). Is it worth it? Evaluating the economic impact of worksite health promotion. *Occupational Medicine, 5*(4), 837–850.

Knox, S. S. (1993). Perception of social support and blood pressure in young men. *Perceptual and Motor Skills, 77*(1), 132–134.

Kohler, C. L., et al. (1993). Use of focus group methodology to develop an asthma self-management program useful for community-based medical practices. *Health Education Quarterly, 20*(3), 421–429.

Kothari, S. (1993). Effects of locus of control on anxiety and achievement-motivation. *Indian Journal of Psychometry and Education, 24*(2), 103–108.

Kottke, J. L., & Schuster, D. H. (1990). Developing tests for measuring Bloom's learning outcomes. *Psychological Reports, 66*(1), 27–32.

Kraiger, K., Ford, J. K., & Salas, E. (1993). Application of cognitive, skill-based, and affective theories of learning outcomes to new methods of training evaluation. *Journal of Applied Psychology, 78*(2), 311–328.

Kronenfeld, J. J. (1993). *Controversial issues in health care policy.* Newbury Park, CA: Sage.

Langwell, K. M. (1990). Structure and performance of health maintenance organizations: A review. *Health Care Financial Review, 12*(1), 71–80.

Larimer, M. E., Palmer, R. S., & Marlatt, G. A. (1999). Relapse prevention: An overview of Marlatt's cognitive-behavioral model. *Alcohol Research and Health, 23*(2), 151–160.

Leviton, L. C., Needleman, C. E., & Shapiro, M. A. (1998). *Confronting public health risks: A decision maker's guide.* Thousand Oaks, CA: Sage.

Maddux, J. E. (1993). Social cognitive models of health and exercise behavior: An introduction and review of conceptual issues. *Journal of Applied Sport Psychology, 5*(2), 116–140.

Mahon, N. E. (1994). Positive health practices and perceived health status in adolescents. *Clinical Nursing Research, 3*(2), 86–101.

McAuley, E., & Shaffer, S. (1993). Affective responses to externally and personally controllable attributions. *Basic and Applied Social Psychology, 14*(4), 475–485.

McGinnis, J. M. (1993). The year 2000 initiative: Implications for comprehensive school health. *Preventive Medicine, 22*(4), 493–498.

Minkler, M., Thompson, M., Bell, J., & Rose, K. (2001). Contributions of community involvement to organizational-level empowerment: The federal Healthy Start experience. *Health Education and Behavior, 28*(6), 783–807.

Mooney, J. P., Burling, T. A., & Hartman, W. M. (1992). The abstinence violation effect and very low calorie diet success. *Addictive Behaviors, 17*(4), 319–324.

Morrison, E. M., & Luft, H. S. (1990). Health maintenance organization environments in the 1980s and beyond. *Health Care Financial Review, 12*(1), 81–90.

Nadakavukaren, A. (2000). *Our global environment* (5th ed). Prospect Heights, IL: Waveland.

Nader, P. R. (1990). The concept of comprehensiveness in the design and implementation of school health programs. *Journal of School Health, 60*(4), 133–137.

Norman, P., & Conner, M. (1993). The role of social cognitive models in predicting attendance at health checks. *Psychology and Health, 8*(6), 447–462.

O'Donnell, M. P., & Harris, J. (1994). *Health promotion in the workplace* (2nd ed.). Albany, NY: Delmar.

Organista, K. C., Munoz, R. F., & Gonzalez, G. (1994). Cognitive-behavioral therapy for depression in low-income and minority medical outpatients: Description of a program and exploratory analyses. *Cognitive Therapy and Research, 18*(3), 241–259.

Petosa, R., & Jackson, K. (1991). Using the Health Belief Model to predict safer sex intentions among adolescents. *Health Education Quarterly, 18*(4), 463–476.

Poole, K., Kumpfer, K., & Pett, M. (2001). The impact of incentive-based worksite health promotion program on modifiable health risk factors. *American Journal of Health Promotion, 16*(1), 21–26.

Rawson, R. A., Obert, J. L., & McCann, M. J. (1993). Relapse prevention strategies in outpatient substance abuse treatment. Special series: Psychological treatment of the addictions. *Psychology of Addictive Behaviors, 7*(2), 85–95.

Reinert, B., Campbell, C., Carver, V., & Range, L. M. (2003). Joys and tribulations of faith-based youth tobacco use prevention: A case study in Mississippi. *Health Promotion Practice, 4*(3), 228–235.

Roberts, L. W., & Clifton, R. A. (1992). Measuring the cognitive domain of the quality of student life: An instrument for faculties of education. *Canadian Journal of Education, 17*(2), 176–191.

Rousseau, C. (1993). Community empowerment: The alternative resources movement in Quebec. *Community Mental Health Journal, 29*(6), 535–546.

Stahl, N. N., & Stahl, R. J. (1991). We can agree after all: Consensus on critical thinking using the Delphi technique. *Roeper Review, 14*(2), 79–88.

Steckler, A. B., Israel, B. A., Dawson, L., & Eng, E. (Eds.). (1993). Community health education. *Health Education Quarterly* (Suppl. 1), S29–S47.

Stephens, R. S., et al. (1994). Testing the abstinence violation effect construct with marijuana cessation. *Addictive Behaviors, 19*(1), 23–32.

Stuart, K., Borland, R., & McMurray, N. (1994). Self-efficacy, locus of control, and smoking cessation. *Addictive Behaviors, 19*(1), 1–12.

Tappe, M. K., & Galer-Unti (2001). Health educators' role in promoting health literacy and advocacy for the 21st century. *Journal of School Health, 71*(10), 477–482.

Tiffany, S. T., & Cepeda-Benito, A. (1994). Long-term behavioral interventions: The key to successful smoking cessation programs. *Health Values, 18*(1), 54–61.

Walker, R. (1993). Modeling and guided practice as components within a comprehensive testicular self-examination educational program for high school males. *Journal of Health Education, 24*(3), 163–167.

Ward, T., Hudson, S. M., & Buliki, C. M. (1993). The abstinence violation effect in bulimia nervosa. *Addictive Behaviors, 18*(6), 672–680.

Weisbrod, R. R., Pirie, P. L., Bracht, N. F., & Elstun, P. (1991). Worksite health promotion in four Midwest cities. *Journal of Community Health, 16*(3), 169–177.

Welch, D. H., Luthans, F., & Sommer, S. M. (1993). Organizational behavior modification goes to Russia: Replicating an experimental analysis across cultures and tasks. *Journal of Organizational Behavior Management, 13*(2), 15–35.

Whiting, S. (1994). A Delphi study to determine defining characteristics of interdependence and as potential nursing diagnoses. *Issues in Mental Health Nursing, 15*(1), 37–47.

Wilkin, D., Hallam, L., & Doggett, M. (1992). *Measures of need and outcome for primary health care.* New York: Oxford University Press.

Williams, T., & Jones, H. (1993). School health education in the European Community. *Journal of School Health, 63*(3), 133–135.

Wilson, B. R., & Spivak, H. (1994). Violence prevention in schools and other community settings: The pediatrician as initiator, educator, collaborator, and advocate. *Pediatrics, 94*(4, pt. 2), 623–630.

Woodward, M., Bolton-Smith, C., & Tunstall Pedoe, H. (1994). Deficient health knowledge, diet, and other lifestyles in smokers: Is a multifactorial approach required? *Preventive Medicine, 23*(3), 354–361.

Xiaojia, G. E., Conger, R. D., Lorenz, F. O., & Simons, R. L. (1994). Parents' stressful life events and adolescent depressed mood. *Journal of Health and Social Behavior, 35*(1), 28–44.

ABOUT THE AUTHORS

Naomi N. Modeste holds a doctor of public health (DrPH) degree and a master of public health (MPH) degree from Loma Linda University School of Public Health, Loma Linda, California. She is a professor in the university's Department of Health Promotion and Education, where she teaches, coordinates the doctoral program in health education and the field practicum for master's students pursuing a degree in health education, mentors students, and conducts research. She has published more than twenty papers in peer-reviewed journals. She has over twenty-five years' experience as a health education administrator in school and community settings in the United States, the Caribbean, and Latin America.

Teri S. Tamayose holds a doctor of education (EdD) degree from Pepperdine University's Graduate School of Education and Psychology and a master of business administration (MBA) degree from Loma Linda University School of Business and Management. She is the director of admissions and academic records for the Loma Linda University School of Public Health and is an assistant professor in the Department of Health Administration. In addition to her administrative duties, she teaches and mentors students in the bachelor of science in public health (BSPH) program, participates in recruitment activities, and has been actively involved with the School of Public Health's student association. She has more than eighteen years of administrative experience in the academic programs of Loma Linda University's Schools of Public Health, Medicine, and Dentistry.